Parkinson's Disease
A Guide for Patient and Family

Parkinson's Disease
A Guide for Patient and Family

Fourth Edition

Roger C. Duvoisin, M.D., F.A.C.P.
William Dow Lovett Professor and Chairman Emeritus
Department of Neurology
The University of Medicine and Dentistry of New Jersey
Robert Wood Johnson Medical School
New Brunswick, New Jersey

Jacob Sage, M.D.
Professor of Neurology
Director, Division of Movement Disorders
Department of Neurology
The University of Medicine and Dentistry of New Jersey
Robert Wood Johnson Medical School
New Brunswick, New Jersey

Lippincott - Raven
PUBLISHERS

Philadelphia • New York

Lippincott-Raven Publishers, 227 East Washington Square, Philadelphia, Pennsylvania 19106

Made in the United States of America.

Library of Congress Cataloging-in-Publication Data

Duvoisin, Roger C., 1927–
    Parkinson s disease: a guide for patient and family / by Roger C. Duvoisin and Jacob Sage.—4th ed.
      p. cm.
    Includes index.
    ISBN 0-7817-0312-3
    1. Parkinsonism. I. Sage, Jacob. II. Title.
    RC382.D94   1995
    616.8'33—dc20   95-4919

9 8 7 6 5 4 3 2 1

CONTENTS

PREFACE

Our knowledge of parkinsonism has advanced rapidly in the 4 years since the Third Edition was issued. So much so, that to bring the book up-to-date required rewriting nearly all the chapters and adding a new chapter to deal with the genetic aspects of Parkinson's disease. My colleague of the past 15 years, Dr. Jacob Sage, has joined me as co-author and took on the task of updating the chapters on drug treatment. The result is a new edition, the fourth since the book was originally published in 1978.

The critical reader will find that important concepts have been markedly changed, some have even been turned upside-down. For example, 5 years ago most "experts" on Parkinson's disease believed that it was due to an environmental factor of some kind. Today, most agree that genetic factors are important and geneticists in many research centers are now actively searching for an underlying gene mutation. At the time of writing the "parkinson" gene remains elusive, but given the current state of the art of molecular DNA analysis it is but a matter of time before it is found. The implications for all parkinsonians and their families are so great that we felt it necessary to devote an entire chapter to this new topic.

At the time of the First Edition, there were still many living patients who had post-encephalitic parkinsonism due to the epidemic of "sleeping sickness" of the 1920s such as the people depicted in Oliver Sacks' book "Awakenings" which was later made into a movie of the same name. But few if any "post-encephalitics" survive today. Post-encephalitic parkinsonism is now only a historical memory preserved in books and old journals. Yet due to its extraordinary nature, the enormous impact it had on our understanding of parkinsonism and the fear that it might some day return, we have retained a shortened account of this remarkable malady. Although levodopa remains after a quarter century by far the most effective drug we have for the treatment of parkinsonism, drug treatment continues to evolve as new drugs and new formulations of older ones are introduced into medical practice. New formulations and ways of administering levodopa continue to develop. The use of the old anticholinergic drugs that were the chief form of treatment for parkinsonism prior to the advent of levodopa has since gradually declined. Today they are used only occasionally. Most have been forgotten and some are no longer available. New secondary drugs designed to enhance or extend the effect of levodopa are under study and some are likely to be in general use very soon.

We updated the chapter on surgical treatment to describe the resurgence of stereotaxic procedures. Stereotaxic brain surgery had largely disappeared after levodopa became generally available about 1970, but in the past few years it has staged a modest comeback due to new technology, an improved understanding of the deep grey matter of the brain (the "basal ganglia"), and the development of magnetic resonance imaging of the brain.

Although it remains an experimental treatment available in only a few medical centers fetal brain cell transplantation continues to attract much attention in the public media. As is often the case, there is much confusion and controversy, in such circumstances, and unrealistic expectations are widespread among patients and their families. Accordingly, we have tried to bring this topic into a sober and balanced perspective.

Finally, we have revised and updated the chapter on historical perspectives, believing that knowing the way in which our present knowledge has evolved over the years greatly adds to our understanding. It is a remarkable story of human achievement of interest in itself.

Roger C. Duvoisin
Jacob Sage

Parkinson's Disease
A Guide for Patient and Family

1

What Is Parkinsonism?

The word *parkinsonism* refers not to a particular disease but to a commonly recognized condition marked by a characteristic set of symptoms. Chief among these are trembling of the limbs, muscular stiffness, and slowness of bodily movement. To this triad may be added a tendency to stand in a stooped posture, to walk with short, shuffling steps, and to speak softly in a rapid, even tone.

The trembling usually affects the hands and feet but sometimes also the lips, tongue, jaw, abdomen, and chest. It tends to occur in the affected hand or foot when it is at rest and to disappear during a movement. For example, trembling ceases in the hand while it reaches out to pick up an object but reappears when the hand is returned to a position of rest. The trembling, or *tremor,* is thus a *resting tremor,* unlike tremors in other disorders.

The muscular stiffness is also of a particular kind. It is called a *plastic rigidity* because a doctor examining an affected person finds a constant, uniform resistance to passive manipulation of the limbs. The affected muscles seem unable to relax and are in a state of contraction even at rest.

The third element of the triad, the slowness of bodily movement, is called *bradykinesia* (from the Greek *brady*, meaning slow, and *kinesis,* meaning movement). It is a very complex phenomenon comprising hesitancy in initiating a new movement or activity, slowness in its execution, and rapid fatiguing. The term bradykinesia also encompasses a lack of spontaneity and a decrease in the performance of automatic movements such as eye blinking, the swing of the arms while walking, expressive gestures of the hands while talking, facial expressive movements, etc., of which we are usually unaware.

THE UNDERLYING DYSFUNCTION

This complex of symptoms that we call parkinsonism reflects the dysfunction of a particular region of the brain—in fact, of a particular system of nerve cells in a center, or nucleus, known as the *substantia nigra.* It is called the substantia nigra (from the Latin, meaning black substance) because it is deeply pigmented; it may be readily noted by the naked eye in specimens of the human brain. Under the microscope pigment granules giving the substantia nigra its dark color can be seen densely packed within the nerve cells. This pigment seems to be chemically similar to the melanin pigment responsible for the color of our skin and eyes, and so it has been called neuromelanin. We do not know its chemical structure precisely, nor what its function may be. However, we believe that this pigment is related in some way to the fact that these nerve cells produce and store a specific chemical substance called *dopamine.* Similar pigment granules are also found in other nerve cells, mainly in cells that produce and store dopamine and the closely related substances adrenaline* and noradrenaline.

The nerve cells of the substantia nigra send long, thin fibers upward to connect with other nerve cells in the deep gray matter of the cerebral hemispheres known as the *corpus striatum* (from the Latin, meaning striate body) (Fig. 1). Dopamine made in the cells of the substantia nigra travels up these fibers to the corpus striatum, where it acts as a chemical messenger transmitting signals to the nerve cells of the striatum. When substantia nigra cells are injured or for some reason cannot produce or store dopamine, a deficiency of dopamine in the striatum results. If the deficiency is sufficiently severe, symptoms of parkinsonism begin to appear. Some neuroscientists have defined parkinsonism in chemical terms as a state of brain dopamine depletion.

A deficiency of brain dopamine can come about in various ways. The nerve cells of the substantia nigra may deteriorate for any of a variety of reasons. They may be injured by a tumor, a stroke, a chemical agent, or a virus infecting the brain (encephalitis). Brain dopamine deficiency can also be caused by certain drugs. A functionally comparable state can be caused by drugs that block the action of dopamine in the striatum. The dopamine is then unable to deliver its chemical message, and the result is the same as when dopamine is deficient. Similarly if the nerve cells of the striatum that normally receive the chemical messenger dopamine lose their ability to receive the message, the effect is the same as when dopamine is absent. This is believed to be the situation in certain disorders. Without going into further detail, it is clear that there are many possible causes of parkinsonism, some more important than others and some very rare.

PARKINSON'S DISEASE

By far the most prevalent type of parkinsonism today is the condition first described by James Parkinson in 1817 in his *Essay on the Shaking Palsy*. It is generally known as Parkinson's disease. It was the first type of parkinsonism to be recognized and remains the prototype against which other types are compared. It is sometimes called *idiopathic parkinsonism* or *paralysis agitans*. The term idiopathic means that the cause is unknown. Paralysis agitans is merely "shaking

---

*Adrenaline is the common name for this substance. Scientists refer to it as epinephrine. Adrenaline and epinephrine are one and the same.

FIG. 1. Left-side view of the human brain showing schematically the substantia nigra and the corpus striatum (*shaded area*) lying deep within the cerebral hemisphere. For simplicity, only one side is shown. Nerve fibers extend upward from the substantia nigra and, dividing into many branches, carry dopamine to all regions of the corpus striatum.

palsy" translated into Latin; it is the official name for the disease in the World Health Organization's International Statistical Classification of Diseases.

The cause of Parkinson's disease is not known. Pathologists classify it as a system degeneration of the brain because specific groups or systems of nerve cells appear to be the target of some morbid process. The disease process seems to select very precisely only certain nerve cell systems. It is clearly not a random thing. The location of the affected cells is such that their deterioration almost certainly cannot be due to poor circulation or to arteriosclerosis. Nor is there any sign of infection or inflammation. Under the microscope, however, pathologists can see an abnormal structure within the affected nerve cells. This structure was first described by Dr. Frederic Lewy in 1908 and so is known as the *Lewy body* (Fig. 2). These bodies are the hallmark of Parkinson's disease. They are not found in other forms of parkinsonism. The selective involvement of certain systems of nerve cells scattered through the brain and spinal cord suggests that an unknown toxin or a deficiency of some undiscovered nutrient may be responsible. Some think that there is merely a premature aging process that affects the cells of the substantia nigra. The truth is that the cause or causes are simply unknown.

The disease rarely affects people under the age of 40 years. The average age of onset seems to be about 60 years. The beginning is usually so insidious and the progression so gradual that it can rarely be dated precisely. Usually the first symp-

FIG. 2. Microscopic view of a Lewy body (*arrow*) within a nerve cell in the substantia nigra of Parkinson's disease patient. To the left is a large clump of neuromelanin granules. It is these granules that give the substantia nigra its black color.

toms noted are, to quote James Parkinson, "a slight sense of weakness, with a proneness to trembling . . . in one of the hands and arms." These symptoms tend to increase very gradually over a period of many years. Indeed progression is so gradual that little if any changes can be seen from one year to the next.

Parkinson's disease is believed to affect about 500,000 people in the United States, or approximately 1% of the population over age 50. It occurs with a similar prevalence in other countries in which good epidemiological studies have been done, and appears in all races of mankind all over the world. It is difficult to make precise comparisons in different countries, however, owing to differences in medical care systems and in statistical methods. Some statistical data are available in England and Wales dating back to the middle of the last century and from various hospitals and university clinics in the United States and several European countries at least as far back as the 1890s. These data suggest that the prevalence of the disease has not changed appreciably over the past century.

Occasionally one encounters a husband and wife who both have the disease, but the incidence of conjugal parkinsonism is less than 2%, approximately what might be expected by chance alone. This is good evidence that the disease is not contagious. Moreover, since it may be presumed that husbands and wives have shared a similar diet and environment for many years before the usual onset of parkinsonism, this observation is also additional evidence that a dietary factor is not likely to be the cause of the disease.

No difference in the incidence of the disease in men versus women has been found. Nor have studies of its incidence in different occupations or socioeconomic groups revealed any special concentration of cases. Parkinson's disease appears to be a democratic disease. The possibility that a virus may be involved in causing Parkinson's disease was once considered an attractive hypothesis. It has been suggested that an unconventional or incomplete virus causing a "slow" viral disease might be responsible. However, thus far no evidence for such a virus has been found.

The possibility that an environmental substance might be a cause of Parkinson's disease has seemed especially attractive in recent years, but despite extensive research no such substance has been found. The relative constancy of the prevalence of the disease over the past century argues against an industrial pollutant, herbicide or insecticide as a causative agent.

It has long been recognized that some Parkinson disease patients have similarly affected relatives. Many patients ask whether their disease is hereditary or runs in families. On casual inquiry about 15 to 25% of patients report that they have an affected relative. On more careful study, however, at least half of patients for whom family information is available turn out to have affected relatives. Families in which cases have occurred over several generations are not uncommon. Thus contrary to the prevailing opinion of only a few years ago, genetic factors are now thought to play an important role in Parkinson's disease. Recent research has increasingly focused on the genetics aspects of Parkinson's disease. These will be more fully described in Chapter 15.

In summary, the cause of Parkinson's disease remains unknown, but recent research suggests that the primary cause may be found in our genes.

DRUG-INDUCED PARKINSONISM

Another common cause of parkinsonism is the drug treatment of mental illness such as schizophrenia. There may be as many cases of drug-induced parkinsonism as there are cases of Parkinson's disease. However, they are almost entirely found among psychiatric patients. The powerful tranquilizing drugs used in treating mental illness block the actions of dopamine in the brain. The resulting disturbance of brain function is essentially the same as that caused by depletion of brain dopamine. The great value of these drugs is that they can tranquilize without causing sedation—that is, without making the patient feel drowsy, groggy, or sleepy. Introduced into medical practice during the mid-1950s, these drugs revolutionized the treatment of mental illness. They quickly displaced the padded cell, strait jackets, water therapy, and the various coma therapies, such as insulin coma, that had previously been the main methods of treatment. However, these drugs also cause a Parkinson-like state that closely mimics Parkinson's disease. Efforts to find an effective major tranquilizer that does not cause parkinsonism have repeatedly met with disappointment. It appears that the tendency of these drugs to cause parkinsonism— blocking dopamine transmission in the brain—is fundamental to their effectiveness in treating mental illness. Some psychiatrists believe that producing a very mild degree of parkinsonism is necessary to obtain good results in their patients. It has been said, partly in jest but with more than a grain of truth, that treatment with the major tranquilizers represents a sort of "chemical strait jacket" more humane and more effective than the old physical methods.

The first of the major tranquilizers was the drug chlorpromazine, known by its proprietary names Thorazine in the United States and Largactil in Europe. Many derivatives of chlorpromazine have been made and are widely used as tranquilizers. These include trifluoperazine (Stelazine), fluphenazine (Permitil, Prolixin), and thioridazine (Mellaril), to cite a few of those in more common use. One drug of this class, prochlorperazine (Compazine), is used mainly to combat nausea and vomiting. These drugs are known collectively as the phenothiazines. A closely related chemical family includes the drug haloperidol (Haldol). This is one of the most potent of the major tranquilizers and quickly induces parkinsonism.

One of the first tranquilizers found capable of causing parkinsonism was the drug reserpine, derived originally from the Indian snakeroot plant *Rauwolfia serpentina*. It was widely used for many years to treat high blood pressure. Although in large doses it can induce a state of parkinsonism, it very rarely does so in the small doses in which it is used to lower the blood pressure in hypertensive patients. Reserpine also causes a condition in animals that resembles parkinsonism, and it has consequently been used in experimental work to help find new treatments for human parkinsonism. Another drug used in treating hypertension, methyldopa (Aldomet), produces a chemical parkinsonism, although this occurs very rarely. Both these drugs induce parkinsonism by causing a depletion of brain dopamine through chemical means. Metoclopramide (Reglan), commonly prescribed for various stomach disorders in the United States, may also induce parkinsonism. It does so in the same way the major tranquilizers do, that is, by blocking the action of dopamine.

All of these forms of drug-induced parkinsonism are reversible. The Parkinson-like state they cause gradually disappears when the patient stops taking the drug or if the dose is simply lowered. It may take several days or perhaps 1 to 2 weeks for the parkinsonism to subside. Rarely it takes more than a month. We have never seen parkinsonism persisting indefinitely after treatment with any of the drugs we have discussed here. There is, however, one chemical agent, *N*-methylphenyl tetrahydropyridine (MPTP) that causes a permanent parkinsonism. It appeared briefly as a contaminant in illicit "street" drugs in 1982, and only a handful of human patients with MPTP parkinsonism are known. MPTP has proved very useful in the laboratory to induce parkinsonism in animals.

POST-ENCEPHALITIC PARKINSONISM

Encephalitis means literally brain inflammation. In common medical usage it refers to brain inflammation due to a virus infection. Parkinsonism occurring as a sequel to a viral infection of the brain is called post-encephalitic, meaning that it came *after* the encephalitis. There is only one kind of encephalitis known to have resulted in chronic progressive parkinsonism. This was a rather unusual type of encephalitis that occurred primarily from 1916–1926 in small epidemics scattered throughout the world. A few sporadic cases were seen during the 1930s and the early 1940s. Only very rare cases have been seen since. The first cases were seen in central Europe in 1915 and 1916, and were studied and described by the Austrian neurologist Constantin von Economo. The condition was thus widely known as *von Economo's encephalitis*. Because it occurred chiefly in small epidemics, it was more generally called *epidemic encephalitis*. It was also called *encephalitis lethargica* because its first symptom was prolonged sleepiness.

In addition to sleepiness, the patients showed various types of strabismus, difficulty in swallowing, and bizarre changes in personality and behavior. Many patients, as many as 40 to 50%, died during the acute, or initial, phase of the illness. The survivors gradually recovered after 6 months or more, with various residual symptoms. Some remained severely crippled, with paralysis, tremors, severe muscle rigidity, marked mental changes, and many other difficulties. Many were thought to have fully recovered, but it was later realized that they too were left with subtle residual symptoms. They looked normal on examination, but their behavior was changed. They remained generally withdrawn and were not able to resume the pattern of their former lives and to return to school or work. They tired easily, had little initiative, and seemed generally passive. They were said to be "neurasthenic." Gradually these survivors also began to show manifestations of parkinsonism. This delayed progressive phase of the illness was called chronic encephalitis and later post-encephalitis. Because the patients had many symptoms similar to those of Parkinson's disease, they were said to have *post-encephalitic parkinsonism*. This peculiar kind of parkinsonism developed in nearly all the survivors sooner or later, with the first symptoms appearing within 3 years in about 80% of them. Eventually all the survivors had some degree of parkinsonism. They also had many other sequelae of their encephalitis that had never been seen in parkinsonism patients before. One of the most remarkable was the repeated occurrence of "visual spells," in which the head and eyes were turned up as if to look at the ceiling for hours at a time. These episodes were called "oculogyric crises." Other unusual sequelae were compulsive tics and rituals that could be so severe as to render otherwise normal-appearing persons incapable of ordinary employment.

The first epidemics of encephalitis lethargica were observed in Europe several years before the great worldwide influenza pandemic of the winter of 1918–1919. There was nevertheless a common tendency to connect post-encephalitic parkinsonism with the flu. No conclusive evidence was ever found that encephalitis lethargica was a consequence of the flu.

Repeated attempts were made to isolate an infectious virus from persons afflicted with this condition, but its cause was never found. Various viruses were recovered, notably the virus herpes simplex, which we now know is responsible for the ordinary cold sore. Initially this virus was thought to be the probable cause, and a vaccine was prepared from it to treat cases of encephalitis lethargica. After many years of research and much effort, a great deal was learned about herpes simplex, but it seemed less and less likely to be the cause of encephalitis lethargica. Looking back at the efforts of the early "microbe hunters" to find the infectious agent of encephalitis lethargica, one can only admire how much was accomplished with tools that by present standards may only be called primitive. Clearly the science of virology was not sufficiently advanced at the time to accomplish the task.

There were a great many patients with this type of parkinsonism during the 1920s and through the 1940s. In fact post-encephalitic parkinsonism was by far the commonest cause of parkinsonism seen by physicians during those years. However, since 1950 new cases of post-encephalitic parkinsonism are very rare. The generation of individuals afflicted by encephalitis lethargica has now passed on, and this particular illness has disappeared from the face of the earth.

No other type of encephalitis has been found to cause anything like the sequelae of encephalitis lethargica. Some symptoms reminiscent of Parkinson's disease are seen rarely during the acute or initial phase of various kinds of encephalitis, but these nearly always disappear during convalescence and never return. Very rarely a few symptoms, such as tremor in one hand, may persist after recovery from some types of encephalitis (Japanese B encephalitis and

Central European tic-borne encephalitis), but these are mild and do not progress over the years, unlike the changes seen in survivors of encephalitis lethargica. Several types of viral encephalitis occur regularly in North America, usually in small, scattered epidemics. These include eastern equine encephalitis, western equine encephalitis, and St. Louis encephalitis. They occur during the summer or early fall and are caused by a virus transmitted to humans and horses by mosquito bite. The viruses responsible for more common illnesses such as measles, chickenpox, shingles (herpes zoster), and the common cold sore (herpes simplex) may also on rare occasion infect the brain and produce encephalitis.

Although all these viruses have been suspected at one time or another of being responsible for some cases of parkinsonism—even for parkinsonism developing many years later—there is no factual evidence to support these suspicions. And that is not for lack of trying. Many studies have been carried out in search of some association between parkinsonism and these viruses, so far with consistently negative results. An example is the long-term follow-up surveys of survivors of western equine encephalitis carried out over a period of many years by Dr. Knox Finley of California and the California Encephalitis Commission. Several cases of Parkinson's disease were found in approximately the number that would have been expected by chance, however.

Extensive studies of antibodies in the blood of Parkinson's disease patients were carried out by Dr. Teresita Elizan at the Mount Sinai Medical School in New York in the 1970s. The presence of antibodies to a specific virus indicates that the person in question has at some previous time been infected by that virus. Over 30 common viruses were studied, including several strains of flu virus. No evidence was found to implicate any of the viruses studied.

ARTERIOSCLEROTIC PARKINSONISM

Elderly persons who have recovered from several minor strokes may be left with some stiffness and slowness, a tendency to walk with short, shuffling steps, and some difficulty speaking clearly. If to these symptoms is added the gently stooped posture common among the elderly, there may be a resemblance to Parkinson's disease. Because the major problem in these patients is impairment of walking, they are said to have "lower-body parkinsonism." They are also said to have "arteriosclerotic parkinsonism."

This is a relatively rare cause of parkinsonism. Arteriosclerosis, or hardening of the arteries as it is popularly called, does not cause true Parkinson's disease. Usually there is little difficulty distinguishing between the two conditions. However, sometimes the distinction may be difficult, and in an individual case even the experts may disagree. This is especially so in patients with a particular type of arteriosclerosis called Binswanger's disease, which primarily affects small cerebral arteries and causes progressive deterioration without overt strokes. Usually these patients have high blood pressure.

Of course everyone over 50 years of age has some degree of arteriosclerosis, and it is always possible to have Parkinson's disease plus some brain dysfunction due to arteriosclerosis, to complicate the situation. Arteriosclerotic changes are not uncommon in patients over age 70.

The differentiation of Parkinson's disease from arteriosclerotic parkinsonism is not just an academic exercise. It has practical value in judging the response to treatment. The symptoms of the latter do not respond to treatment as well as do those of true Parkinson's disease, and the elderly arteriosclerotic patients are more apt to experience side effects of drug treatment.

SYMPTOMATIC PARKINSONISM

A variety of diseases and intoxications can involve the substantia nigra, damage its nerve fibers on their long path to the corpus striatum, or injure the corpus striatum itself and thus cause some degree of parkinsonism. In such cases the parkinsonism is considered to be a symptom of another disease. For example, brain tumors may rarely, if they happen to be in the right place, result in some parkinsonian symptoms. Similarly head injuries, congenital malformations, and various infections, such as tuberculosis or syphilis, on rare occasions cause some degree of parkinsonism.

Certain types of poisoning tend to injure the corpus striatum selectively and may cause some symptoms resembling those of parkinsonism. The best known disorders of this type are carbon monoxide poisoning, and carbon disulfide and manganese intoxication. Victims of these intoxications may recover from prolonged coma with symptoms of diffuse brain damage, including some elements of parkinsonism. Parkinsonism has not resulted from chronic exposure to low levels of carbon monoxide. Manganese intoxication occurs chiefly in workers mining manganese ore. In recent years it has been encountered in Taiwan and Chile but not in North America or Western Europe. Manganese causes damage to the lungs as well as to the nervous system. The damage to the nervous system is extensive, and the symptoms include much more than parkinsonism.

The "punch drunk" state in oldtime boxers who have suffered repeated blows to the head also includes elements of parkinsonism. There is also a case on record of a man who suffered a bullet wound of the brain that destroyed the substantia nigra on one side. Symptoms similar to those of Parkinson's disease developed on the other side of the body and persisted for many years without further progression.

Rarely parkinsonism occurs in adolescents or young adults (juvenile parkinsonism). Some of these cases represent true Parkinson's disease. Others are due to any number of rare hereditary disorders. One of these is a rare condition known as dopa-responsive dystonia, which usually presents in childhood with a disturbance of walking and twisting movements of the feet; parkinsonian symptoms develop later. This condition may be confused with juvenile onset Parkinson's disease. The symptoms are completely controlled by very small doses of levodopa. Unusual cases of Huntington's disease appearing in adolescence may also mimic parkinsonism. Wilson's disease, a rare inborn error of copper metabolism, is another rare cause of juvenile parkinsonism.

PARKINSONISM PLUS

In many chronic progressive disorders of the nervous system, Parkinson symptoms may occur along with some other symptoms reflecting dysfunction of the cerebellum or other parts of the nervous system. These conditions are often called *parkinsonism plus,* the plus referring to symptoms that do not occur in true Parkinson's disease. These are clearly different diseases. The most common of these are progressive supranuclear palsy (PSP) and multiple system atrophy (MSA).

PSP was first described by Drs. Steele, Richardson, and Olszewski in Toronto, Canada, in 1965. In retrospect the condition occurred many years before but had not been recognized. Considered a rarity at first, it is now diagnosed more frequently, and it is the most common form of parkinsonism plus. At first it masquerades as ordinary parkinsonism, but after several years additional symptoms appear. These include a very particular disturbance in eye movements that points to the correct diagnosis.

MSA comprises two conditions that often occur together: olivopontocerebellar atrophy (OPCA) and striatonigral degeneration (SND). These terms merely describe the pattern of atrophy or shrinkage that may be found on anatomical examination of the brain. In some cases of MSA, regulation of blood pressure, control of the urinary bladder, and sexual function are impaired. These patients are said to have Shy–Drager syndrome.

Collectively, MSA and PSP account for about 15 to 20% of all cases of parkinsonism seen in medical practice today. They are often very difficult to distinguish from Parkinson's disease in the initial several years of symptoms.

ALZHEIMER'S DISEASE AND PARKINSONISM

Some patients with Alzheimer's disease may have parkinson symptoms. Occasionally Parkinson's disease and Alzheimer's disease may occur together in the same individual. Such occurrences are thought to be purely coincidental. After all, both are relatively common disorders in the population over age 65, and thus one could expect that some unfortunate individuals would simply by chance suffer both conditions. To complicate matters further, mental impairments similar to those of Alzheimer's disease develop in some patients with Parkinson's disease in which the cerebral cortex is also affected. These cases may be diagnosed and treated as Alzheimer's disease. It is extremely difficult in such cases to distinguish the two conditions. The correct diagnosis may only be made on postmortem examination.

SUMMARY

Parkinson's disease has been known for nearly 180 years. Most authorities believe it is a specific disease. Although its cause is not yet known, it is believed genetic factors play an important role. In addition there are many disorders resembling Parkinson's disease to varying degrees. In some the cause is known. There is also the remarkable fact that several groups of drugs can produce a condition that closely resembles Parkinson's disease, but disappears when the drugs are discontinued.

All these conditions resembling Parkinson's disease are called parkinsonism. Thus there is a post-encephalitic parkinsonism, drug-induced parkinsonism, arteriosclerotic parkinsonism, etc. Most of these forms of parkinsonism share one thing in common with Parkinson's disease: A particular set of nerve cells in a center called the substantia nigra are injured or impaired, with the result that the brain is depleted of a chemical substance known as dopamine.

2

The First Symptoms

So gradual and insidious is the onset of Parkinson's disease that patients can rarely pinpoint the precise date it began. At best they remember when they first became aware of its presence. In many cases the first signs of the disorder appear long before the patient suspects that anything is amiss. Sometimes one can find evidence that the disorder may have begun several or even many years before its symptoms are recognized. For example, on reviewing old home movies or videos, one can see that a patient failed to swing one arm while walking 5 or 6 years before tremor appeared in that arm. Old snapshots may show that the patient began to have a stooped posture many years before anything was suspected.

One of our patients had once consulted a speech therapist because of "mumbling" speech that made his work as a salesman difficult. Eight years later he developed tremor in one hand and consulted a neurologist. Tremor of the hand accompanied by rigidity of the arm as well as a soft, "mumbly" speech were noted on examination. It was then clear that the mumbly speech had in fact been the first manifestation of Parkinson's disease in that patient, but no one suspected the correct diagnosis until the tremor appeared. It is unlikely that even the most observant diagnostician could have found sufficient evidence to make the diagnosis when mumbly speech was the only problem.

Strangely it often happens that the first sign of parkinsonism is noted not by the patient but by someone else. Usually it is someone close to the patient—a spouse, relative, friend, or colleague at work—who notices some change. Perhaps there has been a subtle change in posture, stiffness of one leg when walking, or a new habit such as holding one arm bent at the elbow and close to the body while walking. The patient usually denies that anything is the matter when asked about these things. A colleague may ask: "Is anything wrong with your leg, you seem to be limping?" Or the patient's spouse repeatedly says: "Stand up straight, you're always bent over lately." Friends and family are often surprised that the patient seems unaware of these changes in posture or manner of walking or moving. They may prevail upon the patient to see a doctor. The interview in the doctor's office may go something like this:

Doctor: "Well, what brings you in today?"

Patient: "Nothing, really."

Doctor: "Nothing?"

Patient: "I feel perfectly well. There's nothing the matter with me."

The patient's spouse may then intervene to describe the cause of her concern: "Doctor, there's something wrong with his left leg when he walks."

So the doctor examines the way the patient walks. He may readily recognize the problem, but it often happens that the trouble is not apparent at the moment. Spouses often complain that the patient always looks much better in the doctor's office: "Doctor, if only you could see him when he is at home."

Most likely the doctor sees that something is indeed amiss, but the telltale signs of parkinsonism are usually not yet present at this stage of the disease, and the doctor probably cannot make the diagnosis. Perhaps he orders a few tests: a blood count, the usual battery of blood chemistries, an electrocardiogram, an x-ray of the chest, and a routine analysis of the urine. This battery of tests constituting the usual checkup probably gives normal results. Parkinson's disease patients seem to be a pretty healthy lot, generally speaking, an observation made by many physicians. The experienced doctor probably wants to see the patient again in a month or two or if further problems arise. At this juncture a little "tincture of time," to quote an old medical aphorism, is appropriate. If something really is going on, it should show itself more clearly in due course.

Eventually the patient becomes aware that something is indeed wrong. There may be persistent tiredness, minor aches and pains, or a vague sense of malaise, of just not feeling well. Perhaps the patient feels a lack of energy or a sense of nervousness and irritability. Performance on the job may be declining for no apparent reason. The patient may notice that things once done with ease, without a thought, now require conscious effort. On seeing the patient again and listening to these vague complaints, the doctor can sense that there is a problem even though all the tests done at the previous checkup were normal. He may try to reassure the patient that the tests were all normal. He may urge the patient to get some rest, perhaps take a vacation, and maintain a good diet. He may even prescribe a mild tranquilizer. If the patient seems depressed, the doctor may prescribe treatment with an antidepressant drug and suggest referral to a psychiatrist. Proper treatment of depression usually helps considerably, and so the patient can carry on as usual for some time.

This phase of Parkinson's disease, in which vague, nonspecific symptoms develop, may continue for a long time. Some patients understandably distressed by symptoms no one seems able to explain tend to visit many doctors and clinics in search of an explanation, but the diagnosis is extremely difficult to establish at this point in the evolution of Parkinson's disease. The symptoms do not point to any specific condition. Overwork, lack of sleep, nervousness, depression, arthritis, poor dietary habits, and similar problems are more likely causes of such complaints.

Later, the patient may begin to experience more specific symptoms, such as soreness in one arm, a sense of weakness or "numbness" in one hand, stiffness in one leg, trouble in carrying out some movement, a change in the quality of the voice. There are almost as many initial symptoms as there are patients. Each individual experiences the disorder differently and interprets the experience in his or her own way. Although these more specific complaints indicate to the doctor that something is definitely wrong, there may still be no physical signs to suggest the nature of the problem. Even if a change in facial expression or a tendency to drag one foot slightly when walking or to favor one hand may be noted, the doctor is still unable to diagnose Parkinson's disease. A single finding is not enough to establish the diagnosis, and there is as yet no blood test—or any other kind of test for that matter—that can establish the diagnosis.

The diagnosis can be made with certainty only when the three characteristic signs are present: *tremor, rigidity,* and *bradykinesia.* Tremor is usually the first to appear. Initially it may be minimal. It may be noticed only when the patient is fatigued or under some stress. Some patients feel the tremor for many months before it is visible. If the writing hand is affected, it is common for the tremor to be noted in the patient's handwriting. Every letter tends to show evidence of a very fine tremor. Usually the handwriting is also somewhat small, a phenomenon called *micrographia.* In addition the patient's writing tends to get progressively smaller on the page or even within a paragraph. The doctor may thus ask for a sample of the patient's handwriting to look for these signs. Occasionally tremor appears initially in a foot, and rarely in the lips, tongue, or jaw.

In a small but significant percentage of patients, there is little or no tremor. Rigidity and bradykinesia may then be the first symptoms. The patient may experience only a sense of weakness of a hand or leg. There may be difficulty with fine tasks, such as buttoning up a shirt or tying shoelaces. Patients whose work or hobbies require some degree of manual dexterity may become aware of a loss of ability. In patients who do not have tremor, the diagnosis is more difficult to establish and may not be made until relatively late in the course of illness.

As soon as one of the three characteristic signs is evident, the doctor recognizes that there is some disturbance in the nervous system and, especially if there is tremor, will suspect parkinsonism. Depending on the symptoms, the findings on examination, and the patient's age and general health, the diagnosis of Parkinson's disease may now be evident at a glance. However, often it is not so obvious at first, and many other possibilities cross the doctor's mind.

In many cases the symptoms concentrate on one side of the body. The patient, for example, may complain of weakness of the left arm and leg, and the doctor may have noted some evidence of such weakness on examination. In appearance the patient with such symptoms—walking with some loss of left arm swing and tending to shuffle with the left foot—somewhat resembles a person who has had a mild stroke.

It happens occasionally that patients convey an erroneous impression that their symptoms came on suddenly. One patient, for example, said that he had first noted trouble with his right arm and leg a month previously and that he was now somewhat better. He believed that he had experienced a stroke. However, his wife described a more gradual and remote onset of his difficulties. It seems that the trouble with the arm and leg had been present for at least a year or more. On further questioning, it became clear that what the patient meant was that the trouble had become important enough for him to pay attention to it about a month previously, and that he had not been fully aware of it before that time. It is quite understandable that a patient who recounts that sort of story to his doctor may be suspected of having had a stroke.

Whereas the sudden development of weakness or other symptoms reflecting troubles in the nervous system tends to suggest a stroke, a slow, gradual, progressive development of symptoms suggests the possibility of some progressive trouble in the nervous system, such as a slowly growing tumor. The doctor may have some difficulty in deciding which of these serious possibilities is most likely, especially in patients with no tremor. Even if there is tremor, however, the doctor will want to be sure it is not a stroke or a brain tumor mimicking Parkinson's disease—that it is indeed Parkinson's disease. He or she may order some neurological tests or refer the patient to a neurologist for a consultation.

The popular image of the specialist as an expert who can make the diagnosis of exotic diseases after briefly glancing at the patient is a gross exaggeration. Of course that does happen on occasion—some conditions, though rare, are readily identified when first seen. Parkinson's disease, when fully developed, is easily recognized. The consultant's task is not merely to make the diagnosis or confirm the referring doctor's impressions but to make sure that what seems to be parkinsonism is not something else. There is no need for haste. Parkinson's disease is not an acute illness or life-threatening. There is ample time to allow the consultant to consider the matter as thoroughly as necessary.

The most important element in making a medical diagnosis is the patient's own account of the symptoms—the "history." The history is more important than all the tests modern laboratory technology has made possible. It is even more important than the physical examination itself. The consultant may ask numerous questions in order to gain an idea of the way in which the symptoms developed. Some questions may seem silly or vague, and patients sometimes answer facetiously or try to guess what is in the physician's mind and so give the answers they think the doctor wants to hear. Obviously it is best to answer as directly and accurately as possible. After all, the consultant can make a more accurate diagnosis when given reliable and correct information with which to work.

The neurological examination is a variety of the familiar physical examination one undergoes during an annual checkup or a pre-employment physical. A complete neurological examination can be a time-consuming affair; the routine examination commonly done by practicing neurologists may require 30 to 45 minutes or more, depending on the circumstances. A great deal depends on simple observation: By the time you have walked into the neurologist's office and said "hello," he has already learned a number of important things about you. During the formal examination conducted after completing the history, the neurologist examines the eyes, ears, mouth, tongue, throat, and neck. He inspects and palpates the muscles in all four limbs and tests the strength of the muscles as well as their tone. He uses the reflex hammer not only at the knee but at other places as well: at the elbow, ankle, and maybe the jaw. Every muscle has a reflex. The eye muscles are tested by studying how the eyeballs move when you follow a moving object with the eyes. Your ability to perceive various sensations—such as a pinprick, the touch of a twist of cotton, the vibration of a tuning fork, and others— is tested. The examination of sensory function is an important part of the neurological examination and can reveal some extraordinary things about higher-level function of the nervous system. Posture (sitting and standing), the character of your walk, the manner in which you get out of a chair, and the way in which you put on your clothes at the end of the examination are all observed. Finally the neurologist usually administers some tests of mental function. These are generally simple items, such as a brief test of memory, abstract reasoning, and the ability to do simple calculations. He may ask you to repeat some numbers, spell some words, do some simple subtractions and multiplications, and perhaps interpret some old proverbs. These may seem silly and embarrassing but bear with it. The neurologist is not so much concerned with whether you answer correctly but the way in which you handle the task. It is also important for him to have some basic idea of the quality of your mental response to the ordinary problems we all have to handle every day. Most neurologists also ask for a sample of your handwriting.

The consultant is usually able to make a diagnosis or at least give a general outline of the problem and the measures that may be needed to pinpoint the diagnosis after completing the history and the neurological examination. He may say: "I believe you have Parkinson's disease, but I'd like to carry out certain tests to rule out some other possibilities." Perhaps your own doctor has already ordered these tests, and the consultant will want to review them before reaching a conclusion.

The neurological tests may include an electroencephalogram, a computerized x-ray tomogram (called the CAT or CT scan), or a magnetic resonance imaging (MRI) scan, as well as some blood tests. These tests do not require admission to the hospital in ordinary circumstances and may be done in the hospital outpatient department or a private laboratory. The CT or MRI scan of the head is not necessary but may serve as a screening procedure in some instances. The chances of detecting a significant abnormality are small, but the test is harmless and a normal result is reassuring.

CT and MRI actually show the internal structure of the brain. The CT scan is a type of x-ray procedure, but instead of using photographic film to display the image, a series of images is constructed by a computer from a tremendous number of readings taken by an array of radiation detectors. The patient's head is placed between an x-ray tube and the detectors, both of which are mounted on a moving gantry in such a way that they can rotate about the head. The detectors can make hundreds of readings in precisely controlled positions. From the readings it is possible to calculate the intensity of the radiation at each of hundreds of points inside the head. A vast number of calculations must be done in order to determine the intensity at a sufficient number of points to produce an image. The calculations can be carried out within several minutes by a computer programmed for that purpose, and the computer then displays the image on a television screen. A series of images are normally obtained, and these are usually photographed on instant black and white film for study.

Magnetic resonance imaging (MRI) works on a different physical principle. The subject is placed within the field of a very large and powerful magnet that causes all water molecules to line up parallel to the magnetic force, just as iron filings do in the field of an ordinary toy magnet. In the presence of radio waves, the water molecules release electromagnetic energy that can be detected by an array of special sensors. Images can then be constructed by computer in the same way as in the CT scan. No x-ray radiation is involved in MRI.

CT and MRI scans are useful in studying patients suspected of having Parkinson's disease or related conditions. They have the advantage of being able to detect not only tumors but also the scars of old strokes and changes in the structure of the brain that are characteristic of various disorders that can mimic Parkinson's disease. Thus, for example, they are helpful in distinguishing arteriosclerotic parkinsonism or parkinsonism plus from Parkinson's disease.

The electroencephalogram (EEG) is to the brain what the electrocardiogram (ECG) is to the heart. Small electrodes temporarily attached to the scalp with glue detect electrical activities arising in the brain. The minute currents induced by brain activity in the scalp electrodes are magnified electronically (approximately 100,000 times) by an amplifier much like the amplifier in a high fidelity set. These activities are then recorded on moving paper so the patterns and rhythms can be analyzed. Abnormal patterns of activity occur in the presence of brain tumors, following strokes or other injuries to the brain, in certain drug and chemical intoxications, and in some persons with epileptic seizures. There are usually only minor nonspecific changes in the EEG in Parkinson's disease. Thus a normal test serves as evidence against the possibility of tumor, stroke, or other brain disorders. As a screening procedure, the EEG is harmless to the patient and may reveal valuable information. A normal reading, although not diagnostic, is reassuring.

These several diagnostic procedures are commonly used to evaluate patients with symptoms indicating some disorder in the brain. All the tests are usually normal in cases of Parkinson's disease. The consultant considers the results of these tests, the history of the patient's symptoms, and the findings of the examination of the patient, and then arrives at the best possible diagnosis. Sometimes additional blood tests may be needed. Rarely a case of parkinsonism with no tremor but only a general slowness in all bodily movement resembles a case of hypothyroidism. A few simple blood tests to measure the blood level of thyroid hormone are helpful in this circumstance. Usually the consultant can say, "I believe you have Parkinson's disease," and can advise the patient on treatment. However, occasionally even the consultant, with the benefit of all the tests described, cannot make a diagnosis with certainty. He or she may wish to re-examine the patient in a month or two. This is not an unreasonable request. The consultant may need time to think about the case. Then, too, the passage of time may allow the disease to reveal itself more clearly.

We have both encountered patients that we had to follow for several months or even a year before the diagnosis of Parkinson's disease became clear. One of these patients was a middle-aged woman who for several years had complained of burning pains in her legs while walking. She was thought to have some circulatory disturbance in her legs and was treated with various drugs to improve the circulation, to no avail. She was then noticed to have a mild tremor of the hands. But there was no rigidity, bradykinesia, or other signs of parkinsonism. The tremor was not of the "resting" type, and so one could not say with certainty that she had Parkinson's disease. Two years later there was slight but definite rigidity in the arms and the tremor had changed to a resting tremor. It was then clear that the pains in her legs and the burning sensations were manifestations of Parkinson's disease, and not of poor circulation. These symptoms disappeared on proper treatment of her parkinsonism.

Some physicians believe it best to reassure the patient with very early symptoms of Parkinson's disease that nothing is the matter. They fear that the very name "Parkinson's disease" will frighten and depress the patient, and so they try to reveal the diagnosis slowly or in stages. These physicians usually advise some responsible member of the family or the family doctor of the diagnosis. Sometimes the families join in this conspiracy of silence or insist on it themselves. They will ask the physician not to tell the diagnosis to the patient. "Mother doesn't know she has Parkinson's disease," a concerned daughter or son may say, "Please don't tell her. We don't want her to know."

In rare circumstances there are good reasons for such silence, but in general it is ill-advised. Invariably patients have been hurt and angered by the attempted secrecy. We say "attempted" because in most instances the deception fails. It did, however, prevent the patients from getting answers to their questions. Since the diagnosis could not be admitted, it could not be openly discussed, and the patient could not learn what to expect in the future, what treatment could be given, what the effects of treatment might be, and so on. They knew well enough that something was the matter, so protestations from the family and the doctor that nothing was the matter gave little comfort.

Once the diagnosis of Parkinson's disease is established and other possibilities excluded, the patient and doctor are ready to discuss the prognosis. Predicting the future is at best somewhat chancy, but some discussion about what the patient may expect, how his or her life is likely to be altered, what the treatment may be expected to accomplish, and so on is in order. Precisely what the diagnosis means to a given individual depends greatly of course on the person and the circumstances. Some patients, perhaps thinking of a relative or neighbor who may have had Parkinson's disease, may fear the worst and imagine that they will rapidly become severely invalid. This is of course an exaggerated view. In fact the symptoms in most cases can be kept under good control for many years. Other patients may have a falsely rosy view. They may recall hearing about a new cure for Parkinson's disease or may have read a glowing newspaper account of a new drug treatment and are confident the doctor can make the whole thing go away with a few pills or injections. This is the other extreme.

Clearly it is important for the patient and the family to attain a realistic view of the nature of the disease and the general outlook. Patients should not hesitate to ask their doctor questions. To this end both patient and family must allow the doctor to be as frank as possible.

Many patients spend much time and effort wondering about the origin of their disease. Often they ask if it could have been caused by some undue stress at work or at home, an accident, or some great personal grief. Questions along this line are quite understandable. They reflect the patient's attempt to grasp in some familiar or comprehensible form just what is happening. It is difficult for many to accept that in this age of incredible technical and scientific accomplishment we do not yet know the exact cause of this one disease or how to cure it. It is best to come to terms with this and approach it with a positive attitude. The late Sidney Dorros put it extremely well in the title of his autobiographical account of his encounter with Parkinson's: "accommodation without surrender."

Parkinson's disease cannot yet be cured or prevented, nor do we presently have means of slowing its progression. However, successful treatment can control the symptoms well enough to allow most patients to lead active and independent lives for many years. Meanwhile research continues on many fronts. Indeed we are confident that current research will soon clarify the mechanism of the disease and, in the years ahead, lead us to more effective forms of treatment than are available today, to methods of slowing or even arresting the progress of the disease, and even to methods of cure and prevention.

3

The Classic Triad

TREMOR

Of the three major symptoms of Parkinson's disease—tremor, rigidity, and bradyki-nesia—the most obvious and familiar is tremor. It is usually the first symptom to come to the patient's attention and most commonly brings the patient to a physi-cian. The hand on one side is usually affected; sometimes one foot is involved. Typically the tremor occurs when the affected hand or foot is at rest. The shaking is regular and rhythmic, with a frequency of 5 to 6 beats per second. A simple, small to-and-fro motion of the arm or leg may be all that is obvious. More often there is a complex movement, with slight turning of the forearm and a back-and-forth movement of the thumb and fingers reminiscent of a hand counting coins or of rolling a marble between the thumb and forefinger. For this reason the tremor has been described as "pill-rolling" in quality.

The tremor disappears when the patient is asleep or resting quietly. Thus it may be present only intermittently, and its presence reflects the patient's state of mind. Nervousness, being "under stress," or even the alertness induced by concentrat-ing on a mental task regularly enhances the tremor. The patient may sit home read-ing the newspaper quietly and have no tremor at all until a visitor arrives. It is this aspect of the tremor that patients find socially embarrassing, and many avoid com-pany for this reason.

Patients may feel the tremor even when it is too fine to be noticeable. It may be felt as a quivering or vibrating sensation. Tremor of the musculature of the ab-domen is felt as a vibration or something "quivering inside." Tremor of the di-aphragm or of the chest muscles is sometimes felt as "palpitations," and the pa-tient may erroneously fear that something is the matter with the heart, and so consult a physician for that complaint. Since the tremor can be detected by elec-trocardiography, it may obscure the electrical record of the heartbeat, making it difficult at times to evaluate the heart properly. The electrocardiogram may have to be repeated on another occasion.

Tremor may involve the tongue, lips, and jaw, but rarely does it cause shaking of the head or affect the voice. Tremor may be confined to a very small part (for

example, one finger). Some patients report that their tremor began in the thumb
or index finger!

A characteristic feature of tremor is its variability. It seems to come in bursts
and then subside. The tremor of one part need not be synchronous with that in another. In fact tremor may appear in a hand for a few minutes and then quiet down,
only to appear in the foot for a while. Most patients are able to stop the tremor by
an effort of the will. Many have learned various tricks to stop it. A slight movement or change of posture may arrest the tremor for a while; eventually it reappears, after some minutes or sometimes longer.

Tremor in one hand disappears while the patient is walking if he or she re-
members to swing the arm. It reappears when the patient forgets and allows the
arm to hang idly at the side—as if tremor were a substitute activity. Holding something in the hand can also stop the tremor. One patient always carries a small pack-
age in one hand when out walking. He found that merely holding the small weight
prevents the tremor, which he is anxious to conceal. Many patients attempt to hide
a trembling hand. They stuff the offending hand into a coat pocket, sit on it, or
cover it with a newspaper or some object or even with the other, nontrembling
hand. Embarrassment at having a tremor is very common among Parkinson's disease patients. In contrast persons with "essential tremor," which is usually more
obvious and sometimes strikingly resembles the Parkinson tremor, do not seem
to share this sense of embarrassment quite so often or so markedly. Why one type
of tremor is embarrassing and the other not is not clear.

Patients have told us that they are ashamed to appear ill to their friends or family. Others fear that colleagues at work or their boss might notice the tremor and
draw unfavorable conclusions. Unfortunately there may well be justification for
the fear of letting the boss, or clients, or customers see the tremor. Doctors, lawyers,
accountants, and other professionals with a Parkinson tremor say that their patients or clients seem to lose confidence in them after noticing the tremor. A clothing salesman was fired with the explanation that his tremor would make a poor
impression on customers! On the other hand, many patients fortunate enough to
work in family-owned businesses or to run their own shops have continued their
work successfully for years despite their tremor. There seems to be a need for better education of the public regarding Parkinson's disease.

In the very earliest phases of the disease, tremor sometimes occurs only at infrequent intervals, during periods of great nervous tension. For example, one patient first became aware of a tremor of the hand after an auto accident while trying to jot down the other driver's name, license number, and so on. The tremor
subsided and did not reappear for several years! Understandably the patient asked
if the nervous strain of the accident might have caused Parkinson's disease in his
case. It is not surprising that similar observations led 19th century medical writ-
ers to consider whether fright or "nervous exhaustion" might not indeed be a
causative factor in Parkinson's disease. Now that we know much more about the
organic basis of the symptoms of Parkinson's disease, we recognize that nervous
tension may indeed increase the tremor or bring it out when it is otherwise not

present. In exceptional circumstances it may even reveal the tremor a few months or years before it might otherwise have been noted.

Tremor occurs in many conditions. One that is sometimes confused with Parkinson's disease is *benign essential tremor.* Generally the tremor of this condition occurs when the arms are held outstretched for a moment or during a movement such as reaching for the handle of a teacup. In contrast the tremor of Parkinson's disease occurs at rest. In other words essential tremor is a "postural" or an "action" tremor. The tremor also tends to affect the head, as well as the voice. The head shakes rhythmically up and down as if the patient were constantly nodding "yes" or from side to side in a "no" tremor. However, the distinction based on the relationship of tremor to movement or position is not always so clear-cut. Some Parkinson's disease patients have an action or a postural tremor for several years before a rest tremor develops as well. These patients for a time may be erroneously labeled as having essential tremor.

The major point of difference between these two conditions, however, is that neither rigidity nor bradykinesia occurs in essential tremor. Thus a physician examining a patient who presents with the complaint of tremor looks for other signs as well, especially for bradykinesia and rigidity. Patients with essential tremor tend to write large and fast, whereas Parkinson's disease patients write small and slowly. One can often suspect the diagnosis from a handwriting specimen alone!

RIGIDITY

Patients often complain of a feeling of stiffness, which is perhaps their subjective appreciation of rigidity. Strictly speaking, rigidity is not a symptom the patient feels, but an objective sign that can be appreciated only by another person during physical examination for evidence of resistance to passive motion. A physician takes the patient's arm and gently bends and straightens it a number of times while asking the patient to relax. The physician is looking for resistance to passive motion around the elbow joint. There may also be similar resistance to passive motion at other joints: the wrist, knee, ankle, spine, etc. A persistent resistance to such passive movement with a plastic quality is what we mean by the term *rigidity.* It has a very characteristic feel and cannot be voluntarily imitated by the patient. It differs from the type of resistance to passive motion encountered in spasticity. There is often a regular, jerky quality to the resistance, as if there were a ratchet gear or cogged wheel in the joint being manipulated. Physicians know this as "cogwheel rigidity."

One can also see on looking at "rigid" muscles that they are constantly tensed in a state of sustained contraction when they should be soft and relaxed when not in use. The tightness and firmness of rigid muscles can be felt with the fingers.

The patient may be aware of the muscular rigidity not only as a sense of stiffness but as a tired, aching feeling, persistent soreness, a pain, or a cramp. Thus rigidity of the muscles of the head and neck is often experienced as a headache.

Usually it is felt mainly in the back of the neck, shoulders, back of the head, and temples. Rigidity of the spinal muscles causes back pain (usually low back pain), which is aggravated by the tendency to stand leaning forward. Constantly leaning forward places the spinal muscles under a mechanical strain. Anyone who tries to stand leaning forward slightly in the posture common to many Parkinson's disease patients soon experiences low-back pain. Rigidity of the muscles of the calf and foot is manifested as painful cramps, not unlike the common charley horse provoked by athletic exercise.

Rigidity of the muscles of the chest and shoulder is sometimes felt as chest pain. When this occurs on the left side, the pain may be misinterpreted as the pain of heart disease known as "angina pectoris." One of our patients visited many heart specialists who conducted numerous tests and could find nothing wrong with his heart. When some tremor and rigidity eventually developed in his left hand, the diagnosis of Parkinson's disease could be made, and it became apparent that the chest pain was a symptom of Parkinson's disease. It disappeared after treatment with levodopa.

Aspirin and similar ordinary pain-relieving medications usually do not provide much help for the pain associated with sustained muscle contraction. Physical measures such as heat and massage are often helpful, at least temporarily. The back pain may be relieved by a hot bath, a back rub, or a heating pad applied to the muscles of the back. Massaging the muscles of the neck relieves headache, and kneading the calf muscle may relieve leg cramps. Proper treatment of the parkinsonism gives the best and most lasting relief. Improvement of the posture is also important in alleviating back pain. The pain often disappears immediately when the patient makes the effort to stand erect. A problem here is that the patient soon reverts to a stooped posture and again has back pain. Exercises to improve the posture are thus helpful but must be performed regularly to obtain good results.

BRADYKINESIA

Muscular rigidity slows movement. Some years ago many physicians believed that tremor and rigidity accounted for all the symptoms of Parkinson's disease. Rigidity may indeed impede movement. All movement requires the cooperation of opposing muscles—some relaxing while others contract and vice versa. The failure of an antagonist muscle to relax obviously limits a given movement. Consider a simple movement such as bending the arm (Fig. 3).

The biceps muscle brings about the movement by contracting or shortening; it is the *agonist* in this case. The triceps muscle relaxes and allows itself to be stretched as the arm bends at the elbow, and it is the *antagonist* muscle here. To straighten the arm, the reverse occurs: The triceps contracts and biceps relaxes. Failure of the reciprocal action of these muscles is the essential feature of rigidity; that is, the triceps fails to relax on bending of the arm, and the biceps fails to relax on at-

FIG. 3. Reciprocal action of agonist and antagonist muscles acting in opposing directions across a joint—in this case, the elbow joint.

tempting to straighten the arm. It is the failure of reciprocal relaxation of antagonist muscles that the physician feels as a resistance to passive manipulation of the patient's limbs. The rigidity impedes not only passive movement but active movement willed by the patient as well. It seems readily understandable that rigidity has been blamed for the slowness of movement (bradykinesia) in parkinsonism.

The reality is more complicated. If patients are observed carefully, it can be seen that slowness of movement may occur in the limbs with the least rigidity and that rapid movement can occur even with rigidity. Rare patients are observed who have bradykinesia but no rigidity at all. Thus the two major symptoms do not parallel each other. Physicians once debated this subject at some length. It was the experience with stereotactic brain surgery that finally convinced skeptics of the importance of bradykinesia. Many patients had excellent relief of tremor and rigidity, but in some cases relief of rigidity did not result in a corresponding reversal of bradykinesia. Rigidity was abolished, but good, rapid movement was not necessarily restored.

Physicians are sometimes surprised to see a patient who looks rigid but shows no signs of increased resistance to passive movement, no signs of true rigidity. This misleading appearance of rigidity is due to the complex phenomenon of bradykinesia, or more simply akinesia (literally, absence of movement), a term that refers to both slowness and poverty of movement. When bradykinesia is minimal, it is barely noticeable and may pass for normalcy. Some persons are normally slower in movement than others. Some are pokerfaced quite normally; others are very expressive. Since the range of normalcy is broad, a mildly bradykinetic parkinsonian patient, especially if elderly, is apt to pass for normal. Persons close to the patient, however, may have noticed a change. A man who was formerly quick and vivacious and has now become slow and deliberate may still be within the range of normal to a casual observer, but those who know him well are aware of an appreciable change.

Perhaps one of the most common manifestations of bradykinesia is the loss of automatic movements. These are movements we normally make without being conscious of them. They occur automatically. They include the swing of the arms during walking, eye blinking, swallowing of saliva, expressive movements of the face and hands, minor movements of postural adjustment, and so on.

A normal person who is sitting is not actually perfectly still. The eyes blink spontaneously a number of times a minute. We are usually unaware of this occurrence or pay it little attention. The motor act occurs automatically without our consciously commanding it. Similarly we swallow our saliva several times a minute. We shift our weight from one side to the other, cross our legs, maybe even do little fidgety movements such as tapping the floor with our foot or drumming on the arm of a chair with our fingers. We turn our head and eyes from side to side to survey the scene around us. We clear our throats, nervously cough, rub our necks, scratch here or there. All these movements are done without significant conscious participation. A striking feature of the severely bradykinetic Parkinson patient is that these spontaneous motor acts are done much less frequently than normal. There is thus a poverty of spontaneous movement.

The reduced frequency of eye blink gives the face a staring expression. The eye blink functions as a sort of windshield wiper, removing bits of dust settling on the surface of the eyes. With reduced blinking the cleansing function is less effective and the eyes may become irritated. The eyelids become dry, reddened, and crusted, and the patient may experience a burning feeling in the eyes. Irrigating the eyes with artificial tears or a suitable eyewash several times a day usually alleviates this problem.

The diminished frequency of swallowing allows saliva to pool in the throat. When this is severe, saliva may spill forward in the mouth and pass through the lips, resulting in drooling. It was once thought that Parkinson's disease patients produced abnormal amounts of saliva, but measurements have shown that this is not so. In fact they produce normal amounts but simply do not swallow it at the normal rate. Treatment with anti-Parkinson drugs improves the rate of swallowing and also reduces the volume of saliva produced. The old anticholinergic drugs employed before levodopa was available dried up the saliva. Drooling was controlled but often at the expense of a feeling of dryness of the mouth.

Another class of automatic movements are those associated with walking. Normally one swings the arms while walking, each arm in synchrony with the opposite leg. Also, when turning, one "leads" with the head. The head and eyes turn first, followed by the shoulders, and later the trunk and legs. The bradykinetic patient fails to swing the arms or swings them to a lesser extent and fails to lead with the head on turns. Instead the body turns in one piece.

Bradykinesia is also apparent in more voluntary movements. Here it is seen as a hesitation in initiating an action, then a slowness in the movement, and finally rapid fatigue, which is especially evident in repetitive movements. These features may occur in many kinds of motor acts. For example, if walking is affected, there is a delay in starting to walk. The feet seem glued to the floor. Finally after several false starts, the severely affected patient walks slowly with shuffling steps. The steps become progressively shorter and then walking suddenly stops. Bradykinesia may be demonstrated in an affected hand by asking the patient to tap the knee alternately with the palm of the hand and the back of the hand. After a few false starts, the patient taps satisfactorily if somewhat more slowly than with the other hand. Then the tapping becomes slower, and finally it stops as the patient seems unable to turn his hand over fully.

Common problems caused by bradykinesia include difficulty getting up from a chair, trouble getting out of a car, turning over in bed, and donning a coat or jacket. The activity begins all right but slows down and falters just before it is successfully completed. It is as if the energy required for the activity suddenly fails. Patients sometimes remark that they felt as if their batteries had run down. Other patients feel the bradykinesia as an external force restraining their movement. This is graphically shown in the self-portrait by an artist patient shown in Fig. 4. The patient has drawn ropes shackling her limbs to indicate her subjective experience of bradykinesia. Bradykinesia is also experienced as weakness or fatigue. It seems that the actions rendered difficult by bradykinesia can nonetheless be accomplished by an effort of the will. This may seem fine to the person observing the patient, and one is tempted to encourage the patient by saying, "You see, you can do it all right." To the patient, though, it seems that something that should be done easily and without a thought requires effort and constant attention. One patient complained to me that getting out of a deep, upholstered chair required "a campaign of instruction to every muscle involved."

Another aspect of bradykinesia is a difficulty in doing two things simultaneously and in stopping one activity to start another. This is perhaps just another aspect of the need to concentrate on an ongoing activity to ensure its proper execution. Ordinary activities such as dressing and eating therefore take longer than normal and appear to be done in a deliberate manner.

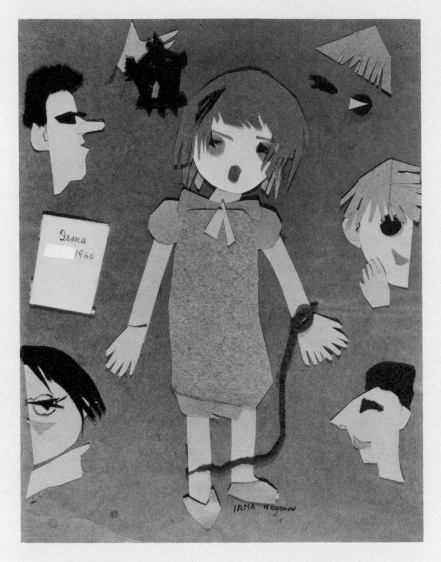

FIG. 4. Self-portrait of parkinsonism in collage by an artist-patient.

Bradykinesia varies considerably from moment to moment and in different circumstances. The patient can carry out an action or movement on one occasion but not on another. The variation is often quite striking in degree. The most striking examples are known as *paradoxical kinesia*.

Every trace of parkinsonism seems to disappear for a brief period. The phenomenon is especially striking in severely affected patients. A chronic invalid who normally can barely walk with assistance suddenly walks down the hall normally, or a very ill patient requiring help to bathe and dress is found to have inexplicably gotten up early and dressed entirely alone. Understandably such variability in performance strains the credulity of the patient's family or attendants. They are apt to refuse a later request for help in some minor task and say: "You did it this morning all by yourself, why can't you do it now?" Alas, the patient cannot do it now and cannot explain why not. This is a common phenomenon in Parkinson's disease, but its mechanism is not known.

The phenomenon itself has been interpreted as evidence that the parts of the nervous system that control and coordinate all motor activity are intact and that they can function normally if properly activated. The basic problem then must be in some defective regulation of those parts of the brain. Here we are at the core of the problem of parkinsonism, for bradykinesia is surely the most important symptom, even though it is not the most obvious one. It is also the most difficult to understand.

Many thoughtful physicians have tried to analyze bradykinesia. One of the great neurologists of the first quarter of this century, Dr. S.A. Kinnier–Wilson, thought of parkinsonian bradykinesia as a sort of "paralysis of the will." He came to this strangely metaphysical speculation because of the sense of effort and fatigue of which his patients complained. Such speculation, however interesting it might seem, does not help very much. What does "will" really mean? What connection is there between the material structure of the brain and a mental attitude or function such as will?

Other physicians saw patients' complaints that "everything becomes an effort" in another light. They argued that action was being blocked by some dysfunction in the brain. Far from the patients' lacking will power, they were in fact forced to rely on will power to overcome some central blocking or inhibiting effect. One eminent neurologist poetically observed that the patients were "condemned to voluntary movement." It has been noted that in general it is the automatic acts of daily life that are most affected by bradykinesia, and learned acts less so. Hence a severely bradykinetic patient may play the piano very well or execute a tap dance.

Professor C. David Marsden, director of the National Hospital for Nervous Diseases, Queen Square, London, has attributed the phenomenon to difficulty in organizing the series of motor "programs" required to carry out a motor "plan" in proper sequence. An apparently simple plan, such as a plan to walk down a hallway and pass through a doorway, requires a large number of changing programs. Typically, bradykinetic patients freeze at the point requiring more complex programs—at the doorway, where additional information regarding the location of the doorway, the number of steps required, and turning must be integrated into a smooth succession.

More recently Professor David Brooks and his colleagues at the Hammersmith Hospital in London have studied the physiology of bradykinesia with an imaging method known as positron emission tomography (PET). They have shown that in normal subjects a small region of the cerebral cortex called the "supplementary motor area" becomes active shortly before a voluntary movement is carried out.

Then the motor cortex becomes active during the movement. In Parkinson's disease patients, the supplementary motor area fails to activate until a dose of levodopa takes effect, restoring activation. Thus the dopamine system directly or indirectly regulates the ability of the cerebral cortex to initiate a movement. Perhaps this is where the "will" to move is located in the brain.

Every kind of activity may be affected by bradykinesia. It is hardly possible to describe all the specific manifestations of bradykinesia here. We can, however, take note of the basic elements of bradykinesia in whatever part of the body or type of activity is affected in a given patient at a given time.

4

A Plethora of Symptoms

There are so many symptoms of Parkinson's disease it is difficult to mention them all in one volume. Many are uncommon or even rare, and few patients ever experience them. Some are fairly common but are more in the nature of nuisances than serious causes of discomfort or disability. Understanding their mechanism and significance renders them innocuous, although, to be frank, symptoms that seem minimal to one patient may be severe and distressing to another.

Many symptoms are only special instances of tremor, rigidity, or bradykinesia. Some of these were discussed in the preceding chapter. We can usually understand the mechanism of these symptoms quite readily, and understanding often reduces them to the level of a nuisance. Other symptoms are not so easily explained. We may simply have no real knowledge of their mechanism except that they are bona fide manifestations of Parkinson's disease.

ACHES AND PAINS

Parkinson's disease does not cause pain that requires a narcotic agent or powerful analgesic drug for relief. A variety of aches and pains do occur, however, and in extreme cases they can be quite distressing. Perhaps the most frequent symptom is an ache or soreness in an arm or leg that seems to be due to tremor and rigidity. The constant motion of tremor may represent a considerable amount of work done by the muscles of the affected limb, and it is understandable that the symptoms of muscle fatigue are occasionally experienced. This may not be the only explanation, however; patients may experience this symptom when tremor and rigidity are barely noticeable but not at times when the tremor is more prominent. A sense of aching soreness may precede the first appearance of tremor by a year or more and then disappear.

A persistent nagging muscle ache may accompany pronounced muscle rigidity. This too may be explained by the considerable work the involved muscles do in sustaining a constant state of contraction. Rigidity in neck muscles is experienced as headache, and in the foot or leg as a cramp. Usually foot cramps occur during the night or on first arising in the morning. Foot cramps during walking are sometimes the initial symptom of parkinsonism. During the cramp the muscles of the foot and calf of the leg are in spasm and cause the toes to bend in a claw-like position. The foot may also turn in at the ankle and sometimes the first toe sticks up. This can be quite uncomfortable, especially inside a leather shoe. Rarely a similar cramp may develop in the hand, usually provoked by tasks requiring fine control such as writing; it has been aptly termed "writer's cramp." Rarely a cramp in the neck muscles may cause wryneck, or "torticollis," a sustained posturing of the head turned to one side. A similar bending of the head forward ("anterocollis") may also occur and, very rarely, a backward bending of the neck ("retrocollis"). These cramps and the resulting abnormal postures are known to neurologists as *dystonia* or *dystonic cramps*. There are of course many causes of dystonia, parkinsonism being only one.

Aching low-back pain is not uncommon in patients who tend to stand slightly stooped over. It is surprising how quickly the pain disappears when the patient stands truly erect or lies down; the pain may be worse in the sitting position because forward inclination of the back may be more marked in that position. Clearly posture, as well as muscle rigidity, plays a role in this complaint. It is reminiscent of arthritis and is often erroneously ascribed to that disorder. However, the usual remedies for arthritis—aspirin, salicylates, ibuprofen, and simple analgesics—do not help, whereas they are quite useful to patients who really have symptoms referable to arthritis.

In addition to these various disagreeable sensations arising in muscles, some patients complain of a feeling of cold or, more often, warmth in some part of the body. It may be a hand, foot, the throat, or one side of the body, or it may seem to be internal, as in the stomach or rectum. One of our patients experienced a feeling of coldness in his left hand for several years. The feeling came and went irregularly; it could be absent weeks at a time and then appear once or twice a day. Wearing a glove alleviated the feeling. Although the hand felt cold to him, its temperature felt completely normal on examination. There was no discernible difference in skin temperature between his two hands! Another patient complained of having cold feet at night for several years. He put on wool socks before going to bed every night, even during the summer. The symptom eventually disappeared.

A feeling of warmth is more common. Some patients experience a burning feeling in one hand or foot. An older woman who has had Parkinson's disease nearly 20 years complained frequently of a burning feeling in her throat and stomach. Extensive examinations failed repeatedly to reveal any cause. She had many x-ray studies of her esophagus and stomach, but there was no ulcer or the slightest hint of inflammation. There was, however, a connection between this symptom and her other symptoms. When for one reason or another her medications failed to take proper effect, her parkinsonism symptoms recurred, heralded by the burning feeling, which simulated heartburn. Tremor, rigidity, and trouble walking soon followed. Adjustment of the medication invariably resulted in disappearance of the burning feeling and improvement of all the other symptoms.

These strange temperature sensations were described more than a hundred years ago as "thermal paresthesias." The medical word *paresthesia* means an abnormal sensation. The cause of these sensations is not known except that they are genuine, albeit uncommon, manifestations of Parkinson's disease. They are not relieved by narcotics. There is no specific treatment for this symptom; generally it responds to treatment of the parkinsonian state as a whole. In one patient spinal anesthesia relieved the burning pain in the legs, but blocks of the nerves in the legs or of the nerve roots by epidural anesthesia had no effect. This suggests that the pain arises in the spinal cord itself.

CHANGES IN POSTURE

Many patients with Parkinson's disease tend to stand in a mildly stooped posture. James Parkinson specifically mentioned this tendency in his introductory definition of *shaking palsy.* He described it as a "propensity to bend the trunk forwards" while standing and walking (Fig. 5). This posture does not develop in

FIG. 5. This Parkinson's disease patient shows the typical "propensity to bend the trunk forwards" while walking, as described by James Parkinson.

all patients, and in many it is barely noticeable. On occasion patients also have a tendency to lean slightly to one side. This is especially noticeable in the sitting position.

Another common change in posture is a tendency to carry one arm bent at the elbow during standing or walking. If the patient makes an effort to swing the arm when walking, the posture disappears. It reappears as soon as the patient forgets to swing the arm. A less common postural change is a tendency to hold the foot turned in slightly. This is usually most evident in the sitting position with the legs at rest. Sometimes it can be noticed during walking.

Characteristically, patients are not aware of these changes in posture. They are sometimes quite surprised when they see evidence of their posture in a mirror or in a reflection in a window. This is not true of all patients, however. Some are acutely aware of the changes in their posture, and it is these patients who are of course in a better position to do something to minimize these postural abnormalities with exercise and by sheer force of will.

PARKINSONIAN SPEECH

Many patients have no change in the character of their speech even after many years of Parkinson's disease, whereas in others the speech may be affected in a characteristic way. Rarely is this the initial symptom. The first change is usually a tendency to speak softly. The patient may have difficulty being understood on the telephone. Strangely, patients are often unaware that their speech is soft and are perplexed that others have difficulty hearing them. A loss of the normal volume of speech may not be troublesome to some patients, whereas it is very important to others. It depends to some extent on the patient's life and work. A teacher, lawyer, actor, or someone who needs to speak or lecture notices the change in speech long before patients in other walks of life.

A patient who was a college professor complained that his speech was not sufficiently loud to be heard in a classroom. When he lectured, the students could not hear him, although his diction was fine. Since he simply could not project his voice anymore, he took a course of speech-training exercises. This helped for a few years, but again the students complained that they could not hear his lectures. Finally he obtained a throat microphone and a public address system. With electronic amplification of his voice, he was able to go on lecturing for many more years.

Another change in the character of speech is a tendency to talk in a steady, measured beat—in a careful, deliberate manner. Neurologists call this "monotone" speech. The natural song and cadence of speech seem to be lost. Some patients speak not only softly and in a monotone but also rapidly. The words are crowded together without the usual pauses between phrases, and the syllables are run together. When these three features appear together, the resulting *soft, monotone, rapid* speech is so characteristic that the doctor should immediately think of Parkinson's disease.

Some patients, however, speak slowly instead of rapidly. Occasionally the voice becomes lower in tone (that is, hoarse), and occasionally higher in pitch. A rare phenomenon is a tendency to repeat a particular syllable in the middle of a word several times. It is similar to stammering yet different in character. The medical term for this is *palilalia*.

All of these changes in speech are improved by effective drug therapy. They may also be helped by speech therapy. The softness of parkinsonian speech is due to a diminished movement of the chest. Normally the chest acts as a bellows, forcing air through the larynx (the voice box) to produce the sound of speech, which is then modulated by the throat, mouth, tongue, and lips to form words (that is, speech). Both rigidity of the chest muscles and bradykinesia affecting the whole action account for the diminished volume of speech. The rapid pace of monotone speech in parkinsonism is more difficult to explain, but essentially the same thing occurs in such other activities as walking, writing, and actions requiring repetitive movements. The tendency to diminished use of facial expressive movements and hand gestures during speech may further hinder the patient's ability to communicate.

SWALLOWING

Akin to the problems of speech are changes in swallowing. The two, however, do not necessarily accompany one another. Swallowing is also a very complex act, although it is performed automatically. In Parkinson's disease the complex sequential pattern of contraction and relaxation of the throat muscles necessary to propel food particles to the rear of the throat and into the esophagus may be slowed. The rate of swallowing is decreased. Consequently eating may become slower and assume a deliberate quality. The patient must wait until the last morsel of food goes down before attempting to swallow the next. Foods seem to be held up at the top of the throat. Liquids and solids are equally difficult to swallow; soft foods seem to go down more readily. Attempts to hurry only make matters worse. Usually it is necessary only to be patient and to eat slowly but steadily.

Slowing of the normal automatic act of swallowing one's saliva results in a pooling of saliva in the mouth and throat. When a large amount is allowed to accumulate, it may spill forward between the lips. The patient is then said to drool. Many patients feel that an excessive amount of saliva is flowing or being produced. However, careful measurements of salivary flow have shown that in fact these individuals form no more saliva than anyone else. Drooling occurs only because the patient fails to swallow at the normal rate. The drug treatment of parkinsonism usually results in both improved swallowing and a reduced production of saliva.

TROUBLE WALKING

Rather characteristic changes in the manner of walking occur in many cases of parkinsonism. The gait is generally less lively, the step shorter, the foot is not

raised to the usual height, and the automatic swing of the arm in time with the opposite leg is diminished or lost. Turns are negotiated slowly, sometimes with hesitation and with the body moving in one piece, whereas normally the head turns
first to be followed by the trunk and then the legs. When walking is more markedly involved, the toe may not be raised off the floor, and the patient consequently
shuffles with one or both feet.

When walking is more severely impaired, several strange things occur. One may
be called "freezing." The patient may be walking along very nicely when suddenly
one foot seems to stick to the floor, firmly glued. After a few seconds it is suddenly loose again. This annoying phenomenon may occur very rarely or frequently.
A curious feature is that freezing tends to occur especially in doorways, while
crossing the street, and on turns. When severe, it may precipitate a fall.

When the freezing phenomenon is prominent, the patient may have difficulty
initiating the act of walking when first arising from a chair or getting out of bed.
A number of very short steps, of an inch or so, are all that can be accomplished,
and then suddenly the patient steps out with a normal step and walks normally
across the room. The neurologist describes this pattern of rapid, short, shuffling
mini-steps as *festination.*

When long runs of festination appear, the patient may lean forward further and
further as the steps become progressively faster and shorter until, after a dozen
steps or so, the patient falls forward unless caught by someone or saved by some
suitable obstacle. Some patients are able to use a cane effectively to stop the forward rush. The entire phenomenon is known as *propulsion.* When it occurs with
backward stepping, it is called *retropulsion.* For example, the patient may make
a few involuntary backward steps when backing out of a closet after hanging up
a coat or when turning around a corner. For patients prone to retropulsion, wearing shoes with high heels may diminish or prevent the backward stepping.

The reasons for these disturbances of walking are not fully understood. Part of
the problem appears to be an impairment of equilibrium. Walking has been described as a sort of controlled falling forward, each step being a response to an
impending fall. A common feature of patients having these problems is a diminished response to an impending fall. The normal responses to an impending fall
are made too late, too slowly, and with movements too small. The normal responses—stepping, flinging the arms, and adjusting the position of the head and
trunk—are normally done very rapidly and instinctively or automatically. Neurologists often test patients in the office for their response to a sudden gentle shove
forward or backward. When suddenly pulled backward by the shoulders, the normal subject simply steps back, flings the arms forward, and bends the head and
trunk forward. The parkinsonian patient with walking problems and poor equilibrium, on the other hand, fails to do these things and instead leans backward
without stepping. If balance is especially poor, retropulsion may result (Fig. 6)—
or propulsion if the patient is pushed forward.

Usually these walking disturbances respond fairly well to proper drug treatment. If necessary, physical therapy with emphasis on gait-training exercises may

FIG. 6. In the phenomenon of retropulsion, the patient is unaware that he is leaning backward, thinking he is standing erect; he is about to step backward involuntarily.

help. Shoes with rubber soles that do not slide easily on the floor may greatly increase the patient's difficulties.

CHANGES IN BOWEL HABITS

Slowness of movement seems to affect the bowels as well as the limbs and all bodily movements generally in parkinsonism. Constipation is a common and recurrent problem for many patients. Several factors may contribute to this. Many patients eat poorly, neglecting roughage and drinking little water. As a result, their stools become small, rough, and hard. This may make bowel movements painful and exacerbate any hemorrhoids that might be present. Constipation is usually only a nuisance, but careful attention to maintaining proper bowel habits fully rewards the little effort required. Rarely, severe constipation may respond only to enemas. Even more rarely, severe constipation is associated with enlargement of the large bowel or colon, called "megacolon." This is due to failure of the nerve cells that regulate the constant activity of the muscles in the bowel. This can result in obstruction requiring a surgical procedure to correct the problem.

IRRITABLE BLADDERS

The normal reflex mechanism for emptying the bladder may be overactive in Parkinson's disease patients. The reflex activates the detrusor muscle in the bladder wall that contracts to shrink the bladder and expel its content of urine. In Parkinson's disease, the reflex may be activated when the bladder is only partly filled. Urologists call this "detrusor hyperreflexia." The patients experience a sense of urgency to empty the bladder as soon as possible. This "urinary urgency" is not uncommon. It is often more marked at night. It is relieved by various drugs with anticholinergic properties. Urologists commonly prescribe oxybutynin chloride (Ditropan).

Less frequently there may be some sluggishness of the bladder musculature so that urination may also be slowed. There may be difficulty in properly emptying the urinary bladder, and the patient may thus have to void again after a short time. Sometimes the patient allows the bladder to overfill, and then suddenly there is an overwhelming urgency to void right away. This is especially annoying at night, for it may necessitate getting up several times. Serious disturbance of bladder function is rare in Parkinson's disease. Should it occur, some other problem should be suspected, such as enlargement of the prostate gland in males or infection of the bladder or a "dropped" bladder in females.

SEXUAL DYSFUNCTION

Human sexual function is complex and intertwined with every aspect of life. It is a many-splendored thing, but it is also very intimate and personal and thus difficult to discuss with a stranger, even a physician. Perhaps this is why few patients complain of sexual dysfunction and why little is known of sexual problems in parkinsonism. Unfortunately there have been few systematic studies of the problem.

The nervous system is involved in sexual activity at every level, from the highest to the lowest. Consequently the nervous control of sexual function is susceptible to disruption at many points. At the highest level psychological factors profoundly affect sexual behavior. For example, depression, anxiety, and frustration provoked by the very fact of being ill may sharply curtail libido. This is a common reason for sexual difficulties in many chronic disorders. Libido may be selectively impaired in parkinsonism by the disease process itself. Dopamine nerve cell systems in the brain seem to play some role in regulating libido. Patients have been described who have parkinsonism, loss of the sense of smell, and decreased libido. All three were improved by levodopa treatment. Although this combination of symptoms has not been systematically studied in Parkinson's disease patients, clinical experience suggests that it does occur in a small but significant number. The improvement of libido on levodopa treatment has been well-documented (see Chapter 7). It may be partial, satisfactory, or perhaps sometimes excessive. Spouses have occasionally complained of exaggerated libido in patients when levodopa treatment is first undertaken.

Rarely the nervous system is affected at a lower level, and the nerves directly controlling the sexual organs may be involved. In the male the result is difficulty in maintaining an erection and delayed ejaculation. Comparable problems presumably may arise in female patients, but so far no evidence on the subject is available. These difficulties are often accompanied by other manifestations of disturbance in the nerves controlling vegetative functions, notably, loss of sweating in the legs and impaired control of blood pressure, the urinary bladder, and the bowel. This complex of symptoms develops mainly in some of the atypical forms of parkinsonism called parkinsonism plus. Indeed impotence without loss of libido may be the initial symptom. Several of our patients experienced this phenomenon for several years before any sign of parkinsonism was evident. They had sought help at clinics specializing in the treatment of sexual dysfunction, to no avail. Unfortunately this type of difficulty is not helped by levodopa. Urologists can help such patients with prosthetic devices and by various medications.

Limitations of bodily movement imposed by rigidity and bradykinesia may cause problems simply by complicating the mechanical aspects of lovemaking. For example, slowness in turning over in bed may make it difficult for an affected male partner to assume a good position for foreplay or coitus. Rigidity and bradykinesia may hinder the pelvic movements necessary for coitus. Some accommodation to these difficulties can be made with some forethought and the assistance of an understanding spouse, but they nevertheless deprive the patient and spouse of the natural spontaneity of normal sexual activity. Improvement of rigidity and bradykinesia with levodopa treatment restore normal sexual activity, chiefly by removing these mechanical impediments.

Many commonly used drugs—notably tranquilizers, antidepressants, muscle relaxers, and simple sedative and sleep medications—may impair sexual function. Drugs used in the treatment of hypertension and the drugs recently introduced for the treatment of benign hypertrophy of the prostate gland in men can also impair sexual function. The anticholinergic anti-Parkinson drugs may also do this to some extent, at least in some patients. Usually these drug effects result in delayed ejaculation and impairment of erection. Thus if a sudden change in sexual function has occurred, it is well to consider whether it followed a change in drug treatment.

Many patients are afraid to discuss their sexual problems with their physicians (and vice versa). They tend to accept them as inevitable accompaniments of their condition or as a natural result of aging. But such may not be the case. Sexual dysfunction may be secondary to drug therapy or may result from an unrelated problem. Awareness of a problem may alert the physician to avoid certain drugs in planning treatment. We urge patients and their spouses to overcome their natural reticence and freely discuss sexual dysfunctions with their doctors. In recent years urologists have developed specific treatments for male sexual dysfunction. These have proved helpful in some of our patients.

LOW BLOOD PRESSURE

In most patients blood pressure is quite normal. Indeed in our experience hypertension occurs less frequently among Parkinson patients than among other persons of the same age. However, a small number of patients may have low blood pressure. The sympathetic nerves that regulate the heart and blood vessels and maintain blood pressure are known to be affected in Parkinson's disease. If the involvement is sufficiently severe, low blood pressure may result, especially when the patient stands up. That is, the pressure may be normal when the patient is lying down or sitting but drops to a low level when the patient stands up. For that reason it is referred to as "postural or orthostatic hypotension."

It is very rare for Parkinson's disease patients to be aware of this low blood pressure, and it is not often recognized because blood pressure is usually measured in the sitting position only. However, if the blood pressure is sufficiently low, patients may experience symptoms of weakness, faintness, dizziness, or light-headedness on standing or walking, especially when first arising after sitting or lying for a time. The tendency to postural hypotension is exaggerated by drug treatment. It is usually easily controlled by various measures (see Chapter 7).

SWELLING OF THE FEET

Swelling of the feet sometimes occurs, usually appearing first and to a more marked degree on the side of the body where the first symptoms of parkinsonism had appeared years earlier. Usually this occurs only in patients with a significant amount of bradykinesia. It seems to be due to diminished movement of the affected leg. The circulatory system relies on the effect of movement of the legs and contractions of the leg muscles to propel the blood in the veins upward toward the heart. If there is little motion, as in the patient who sits still all day, the veins in the legs become congested; some fluid then leaks out and accumulates in the tissues, chiefly in the feet and ankles.

This fluid accumulation is called "edema." It tends to diminish overnight and to increase during the day. If one presses down firmly on the skin of the ankle with the tip of a finger, it produces a small pit or depression that persists for some time. Physicians often search for this sign of edema when examining patients whose ankles seem swollen.

The swelling itself is usually mild in Parkinson patients and has no sinister significance. Sometimes patients think their legs are heavy and ascribe their difficulty in walking to the swelling. Of course their swollen feet have nothing to do with their problems in walking. Occasionally the swelling makes it difficult to put on tight shoes, but otherwise the problem is chiefly a matter of appearance, that is, "cosmetic." The edema usually subsides after proper treatment of the parkinsonism and as the patient becomes more mobile and moves the legs more vigorously. Sometimes additional measures are employed, such as use of a diuretic drug.

SEBORRHEA

Excessive discharge of the oily secretion of the sebaceous glands of the skin commonly occurs in Parkinson's disease. The skin of the forehead, the face at the sides of the nose, and the scalp are particularly affected. The forehead appears oily or greasy all the time but more so in warm weather. The oily discharge may be irritating to the skin and cause redness, itching, and scaling. On the scalp the scaling is recognized as dandruff. When the irritation is sufficiently annoying, it may be termed *seborrheic dermatitis*. This is a common skin disorder that occurs in many people who do not have Parkinson's disease or any other disorder of the nervous system. Dandruff alone is even more common. The various treatments (chiefly detergents and soothing lotions) commonly used for dandruff and seborrheic dermatitis may be used as effectively in Parkinson patients as in others.

EXCESSIVE SWEATING

Excessive sweating is another common manifestation of Parkinson's disease. It may affect one side of the body or even just one area, but it is usually generalized. The excessive sweating tends to occur in irregular bursts. It seems that the sweat glands are somehow poorly controlled and may respond to normal stimuli in an exaggerated manner. The tendency to excessive sweating is usually greatly reduced by treatment of parkinsonism. The mechanism is not understood.

CONJUNCTIVITIS

The decreased frequency of eye blink may result in the annoying symptom of burning or itching of the eyes. The reason is that the normal "windshield wiper" function of the eyelids is not being carried out with the normal frequency. Thus dust particles, grit, smoke, and other irritants that are normally swept away with a blink are allowed to remain for an unduly long time. Consequently the white of the eyes and the eyelids may become irritated. The eyes appear bloodshot, and crusts form on the edges of the lids. Irrigating the eyes with artificial tear solutions usually relieves these symptoms quite readily.

HANDWRITING IN PARKINSONISM

Characteristic changes in handwriting that occur in Parkinson's disease may be of diagnostic value to the physician and a nuisance to the patient. The handwrit-

This is a sample of my beautiful handwriting

FIG. 7. Sample of handwriting showing micrographia. If one looks carefully with a magnifying glass, tremor is evident; look especially at the "f" in beautiful.

ing tends to get smaller. The letters are well formed but get progressively smaller as the patient continues to write; at the end the letters may be so small as to be difficult to read. However, if one looks at the writing with a magnifying glass, the letters still seem well formed. This pattern may not be evident when the patient writes only a few words or a signature, but if samples of the signature going back several years are examined, a change is often evident. The tendency to write small is called *micrographia*. In addition if one looks closely, tremor may be evident in the writing in the form of very small squiggles in each letter (Fig. 7).

Effective drug treatment of parkinsonism produces marked changes in handwriting. It may become normal again, or it may be overcorrected so that now the patient writes in an unusually bold, large hand with extravagant flourishes. This is characteristic of the handwriting of patients with chorea and seems to parallel the appearance of drug-induced chorea (a subject discussed in Chapter 7).

VISUAL PROBLEMS

Occasionally patients with longstanding Parkinson's disease complain of difficulty reading. They consult an ophthalmologist or an optometrist but are told their eyes are normal. They may need a new set of reading glasses, but aside from this, no ocular abnormality is found. Tests of visual acuity are normal. Sometimes patients are advised that the medication given to treat their parkinsonism may be the cause of their visual problem. This is, however, usually not the case. The oculists are simply unable to explain the patient's complaint.

One reason for difficulty reading is that the eyes do not move properly to scan a line of print. The eyes move in an irregular, jerky manner—slowing here, jumping ahead there—so the patient has to work hard to make out the sequence of letters and words. Then, having reached the end of the printed line, the patient has difficulty moving the eyes back to the left and down one line to find the beginning of the next line. Reading thus becomes a laborious task, and the patient soon tires of it. The problem is not in the eyesight itself. The optical properties of the eye have not changed. The problem is impaired coordination of the muscles that move the eyeballs from side to side and up and down. That this is indeed the problem can usually be ascertained with a little thought and careful analysis. There seems to be an analogy between the disturbances in walking and those in eye movement in parkinsonism. The eyes festinate, freeze, and travel slowly across the printed page while reading.

A rare phenomenon, ocular lateropulsion, may occur in which the gaze tends to drift involuntarily to one side so the patient has difficulty directing vision to the desired point. This seems analogous to the disturbance in equilibrium and walking called lateropulsion in which the patient tends to veer to one side.

These disturbances in the coordination of the muscles that move the eyeballs are usually greatly benefited by levodopa therapy. However, they may not always be completely alleviated. Even so, marked impairment of eye movement is distinctly unusual in Parkinson's disease and, if unresponsive to treatment, suggests that a diagnostic reevaluation is in order. If there is obvious impairment of eye movement, the diagnosis may need revision or else some other eye problem may have developed.

Very occasionally a patient with Parkinson's disease may experience double vision. The patient sees two separate images of the world about him, each separate but overlapping the other, somewhat like the split image in a camera range finder when the lens is out of focus. This is due to the fact that both eyes are not looking at precisely the same point. This ocular phenomenon was common in the postencephalitic form of parkinsonism but may also occur, although rarely, in Parkinson's disease and other forms of parkinsonism. The problem is probably in the nerve cells that control the muscles moving the eyeballs. A curious feature is that the double vision tends to fluctuate. It may be present on some occasions, absent on others, and may vary during the day from minimal to marked. Spectacles with special prisms may correct the double vision. However, due to the variability of the phenomenon, some patients are helped by prisms but others are not. Usually in time the patient becomes tolerant of the double vision. The brain learns to ignore one of the images, and double vision is no longer experienced, even though it can be demonstrated by appropriate testing of the eyes.

There seems also to be a more subtle problem with vision in some patients that may be described as "an impairment of visual perception," that is, there is some problem in the interpretation of the image cast on the retina by the lens system of the eye. The nature and significance of this dysfunction is not understood and is the subject of current research. It was recently discovered that the retina has a special group of nerve cells that contain dopamine. The possibility arises that the retinal cells may be depleted of dopamine in Parkinson's disease. Whether such a depletion does in fact occur is not yet known, but it could explain some of the more subtle disturbances of vision that occur.

If one looks at a pattern of alternating light and dark bars or at a flashing light, changes occur in the electrical activity of the brain that can be detected by electrodes placed on the back of the head over the part of the brain concerned with vision. These may be seen on the ordinary electroencephalogram (EEG), but computer analysis of the EEG is needed to sort out the visual effect from other electrical activities. The result is a characteristic pattern of activity called the "visual evoked potential" (VEP). The VEP is frequently abnormal in patients with Parkinson's disease. It is delayed and disorganized. The significance of this finding is uncertain, but it might be caused by depletion of retinal dopamine. It is interesting that the VEP returns toward normal after treatment with levodopa. Although many patients have an abnormal VEP, very few are aware of any impairment of vision, and they carry out ordinary activities of daily living without any evidence of defective vision or disturbance of visual perception.

5

Principles of Treatment

The desire to take medicine is perhaps the greatest feature which distinguishes man from animals.
— Sir William Osler

Over the long run the patients who are the most successful in dealing with Parkinson's disease are those who enjoy a good working relationship with their physicians and families. The treatment of parkinsonism is necessarily more than the relief of specific symptoms. It is a cooperative undertaking, a joint enterprise of the patient, family, and doctor. Working together over the years, they seek to achieve not only the most satisfactory control of troublesome symptoms but also to make living with the disease as effective and successful as possible. Needless to say, the support and love of a concerned spouse and of the family as a whole make a great difference.

Ideally it is best to continue with one physician, preferably the family doctor or an internist who can assume overall responsibility for medical care, and to rely on specialist consultants when the primary physician needs their help for diagnosis, for specific advice regarding treatment, and for special problems that may arise from time to time. However, in the real world the primary care physician, whether trained in family medicine or internal medicine, has had little training in neurology and is unlikely to be familiar with the complexities of Parkinson's disease and the drugs available for its treatment. It has been estimated that the average primary care physician sees fewer than three Parkinson patients a year—not enough to maintain familiarity with the condition. Thus it is best for the patient to visit a neurologist, not only to confirm the diagnosis at the outset and initiate treatment but also to follow the patient's progress over the years. We have found that follow-up visits every 3 to 6 months are adequate for most patients.

In many medical centers there are groups of neurologists who specialize in the management of Parkinson's disease and related disorders. These are often called "movement disorders centers." Patients with unusual symptoms or those who have not responded well to the usual treatment programs may be well advised to visit such a center.

Continuity of medical care with regular visits and periodic checkup examinations is of great importance in a chronic disorder such as Parkinson's disease. It is a deplorable waste of time for patients to shop about from one doctor to another looking for a better or a new treatment without giving each new doctor sufficient time to become acquainted with and to learn the patient's individual reactions to the various treatments available. There are no secret treatments known only to one doctor or available only at a certain clinic or hospital.

There is no curative treatment for Parkinson's disease at present. Several years ago the DATATOP (Deprenyl and Tocopherol Antioxidant Therapy of Parkinsonism) study suggested that treatment with the drug selegiline (Eldepryl) (also known generically as deprenyl) might retard progression of the disease, at least in the early stages in newly diagnosed cases. Unfortunately the preliminary finding was not confirmed on further study or in other similar studies performed in Europe. However, the DATATOP study did conclusively show that vitamin E had no protective effect in the disease.

Although no curative or protective therapy is yet available, there are a number of drugs that can substantially relieve the symptoms for long periods of time. The most effective and most commonly used is levodopa. First introduced in the 1960s, it remains to the present time the best and safest drug available for the treatment of parkinsonism. It is nearly always used in a formulation combining it with either carbidopa (Sinemet) or benserazide (Madopar) to enhance its activity and prevent some of the side effects, especially nausea. It is commonly used as the initial treatment of Parkinson's disease. The symptoms can be so well controlled that progression of the underlying disease may be effectively masked for many years. Patients often forget what having parkinsonism is like. Unfortunately if they discontinue treatment, the symptoms recur. Thus treatment must be continued indefinitely—essentially for the remainder of the patient's life or until someone discovers a better treatment or a cure. Additional drugs may be used to control specific symptoms not relieved by levodopa. Over the years variations in the dosage and the daily schedule of medication or change to a different formulation (for example a slow-release preparation) may be needed to maintain the best results, but levodopa remains the mainstay of treatment in the great majority of patients.

Physical therapy or informal exercise is often helpful and sometimes necessary. There is no specific dietary or vitamin therapy, although attention to one's general health and thus a proper diet is as beneficial to Parkinson patients as to anyone else. Brain surgery to relieve tremor and rigidity was largely abandoned after the introduction of levodopa 25 years ago. It continued to be performed to a limited extent in a few centers. Recently there has been renewed interest in brain surgery, specifically in an operation called "pallidotomy." This procedure is useful in alleviating certain symptoms. An important element of treatment is the interpretation of symptoms, as well as the advice and reassurance that an understanding and knowledgeable doctor can provide. It is essential to adjust one's life to the reality of the disease. All these things are important, but in the final analysis the cornerstone of effective treatment is the proper use of various drugs.

It is important that patients know something about their medication. They should understand why they are taking it and what results may be expected. They should be aware of the major common side effects and how we can deal with them. With such knowledge patients can better cooperate with their doctor and so treatment can be more effective. However, treatment should be left to the physician. Self-treatment often leads to insuperable difficulties. Even patients who are themselves physicians should leave the treatment to another. An old aphorism has it that the doctor who treats himself has a fool for a patient and an incompetent for a physician. The wisdom of this familiar saying applies to all patients. Even if you do know something about the disease and its treatment, you cannot do a good job treating yourself. It is too difficult to judge objectively your own responses to treatment and to observe accurately your own symptoms.

Simply put, the drugs currently available for the treatment of parkinsonism act either by replenishing brain dopamine, mimicking the action of dopamine, or by modifying the function of the brain in such a way as to compensate in some degree for the deficiency of brain dopamine. Dopamine is only one of many chemical messengers in the brain. Another messenger substance bears the chemical name *acetylcholine*. It is a very important substance. Indeed there is much more acetylcholine in the brain than dopamine. It appears to be the chemical messenger for many nerve cell systems throughout the brain and is present in large amounts in the corpus striatum. Unlike dopamine, acetylcholine is not deficient in parkinsonism. On the contrary there appears to be a reciprocal, seesaw relationship between these two messengers and their respective nerve cell systems. Dopamine is believed to act to restrain acetylcholine nerve cells. Dopamine deficiency in parkinsonism thus removes a restraining influence on acetylcholine nerve cells, and their unrestrained and consequently improperly regulated activity contributes in some manner to the various symptoms. Drugs that block or inhibit the action of acetylcholine tend to ameliorate the symptoms, whereas drugs that act by enhancing or imitating the action of acetylcholine cause an increase of parkinsonian symptoms. The opposite occurs in the case of dopamine. Drugs that block the function of the dopamine nerve cells produce the disorder or make parkinsonism worse, whereas drugs that enhance these nerve cells relieve the symptoms.

The drugs useful in the treatment of parkinsonism can be understood in terms of this seesaw relationship of dopamine and acetylcholine. On the one hand are the drugs that block the action of acetylcholine; these are the *anticholinergic drugs*. On the other hand are the drugs that enhance or imitate the action of dopamine; we will call these *dopaminergic* drugs. A very large number of drugs can block acetylcholine, and a few of these are recognized as anti-Parkinson drugs. Their overall efficacy is limited. On average they can reduce the intensity of the symptoms of Parkinson's disease approximately 20 to 25%. They can completely abolish drug-induced parkinsonism. Several types of drugs can enhance the function of dopamine nerve cell systems. Perhaps one of the most familiar is amphetamine. However, amphetamine and its numerous cousins have very little effect in Parkinson's disease. Since amphetamines work indirectly by causing dopamine nerve cells to release dopamine, they might reasonably be expected to be ineffective when there is a deficiency of dopamine, and thus the poor effect of amphetamines in parkinsonism need not be surprising.

The most effective way of improving the function of the "sick" dopamine nerve cells is to replenish the depleted stores of dopamine. This is most easily accomplished by feeding patients the precursor substance L-dopa, which is converted in the brain to dopamine. (L-dopa is the naturally occurring substance that is the active ingredient of the generic drug levodopa; for the sake of simplicity levodopa will be used when referring here to this brain chemical; see Chapter 7.) Drugs that mimic the action of dopamine are also useful in treating parkinsonism. They offer the theoretical advantage of not having to be converted in the brain to the active substance; they act directly on the dopamine receptors in the corpus striatum, in effect imitating or substituting for dopamine. They are called "dopamine-receptor agonists." They are less effective than levodopa but more effective than the anticholinergics.

One drug widely used in treating parkinsonism, amantadine (Symmetrel), is difficult to classify because we are not sure just how it works. It does not seem to have direct acetylcholine-blocking properties. It is thought by some researchers to act on the dopaminergic system, but this is unlikely in the doses used in humans. Recent evidence suggests that amantadine possesses indirect anticholinergic properties. Its side effects and the symptoms of overdosage with amantadine are similar to those of the ordinary anticholinergic drugs.

A quarter century after it was introduced, levodopa remains the most effective agent available for the treatment of Parkinson's disease and most types of parkinsonism; the exception to this is that it does not reverse parkinsonism induced by the major tranquilizing drugs. We prefer to initiate treatment with levodopa in early or mild cases of Parkinson's disease. Some neurologists, however, prefer to initiate treatment with a dopamine-receptor agonist and occasionally with one of the anticholinergic drugs or with amantadine, reserving levodopa for more severe cases or for use at a later date. They delay the use of levodopa in the hope that doing so will delay the development of some of the complications of long-term treatment such as dyskinesias and the on–off effect. The evidence presented in support of this view seems less persuasive to us than the contrary evidence presented by Drs. Charles Markham and Shirley Diamond of the University of California in Los Angeles. Their long-term follow-up studies indicated that patients who began levodopa treatment early in the course of their illness fared better 17 to 20 years later than those who started treatment later. It is difficult to make hard and fast rules that would be applicable to all cases about which course to follow. Despite some persisting controversy over when to begin treatment with levodopa, there is general agreement among the experts that it should be started when the patient has sufficient symptoms to affect life style or employment. The treating doctor must evaluate each case in the light of his or her personal experience, and the doctor and the patient should jointly decide which way to go after discussing the pros and cons.

SIDE EFFECTS

Whichever drugs or combination of drugs is employed, certain general patterns of response may be expected. Much depends on the precise dosage and timing of the drugs taken. With proper care and diligence on the part of both patient and doctor, very good results can be achieved in most cases. The relief of symptoms can be striking. Usually, however, some side effects may have to be accepted in exchange for the benefits. Naturally some patients are more sensitive to the drugs than others. Some side effects are only mildly annoying, whereas others can be quite distressing. Generally the higher the dose, the greater are both the benefits and the side effects. The goal of treatment is to find the best possible compromise between the desired effects—that is, relief of parkinsonism—and the undesired or side effects.

We should distinguish side effects from adverse effects. Side effects are normal effects of a drug proportional to the dosage. Individuals vary considerably in responsiveness, and thus a given effect may occur at a low dose in some persons and at a high dose in another. In any single person, however, effects become greater as the dose increases. Some effects are desirable but only up to a point. After that they are undesired, or side, effects. For example, the reduction in salivary flow by anticholinergic drugs may be a desirable effect in a patient with excessive flow of saliva, but at a higher dose or in another patient, annoying dryness of the mouth may occur. This is then a side effect. Lowering the dose can reduce the effect to a desirable effect. In the same sense drunkenness is a side effect of whiskey. One glass may produce a pleasant state of mind but a higher dose produces the side effect of intoxication.

Side effects can be serious, even life-threatening, with whiskey as well as with the various anti-Parkinson drugs. Thus careful adjustments of dosage is necessary to obtain the balance between desired and undesired effects best suited to each patient. To strike the right balance is not always an easy task. It cannot be done by the patient. It must be done by another person who can see the patient objectively, preferably a person who knows something about the chemistry of the drug, its toxicity, its interaction with other drugs, and management of its side effects. In short the regulation as well as the prescribing of drugs should be left to the physician. In our experience the patients who derive the best results from drug treatment are generally those who follow their prescribed regimen consistently and precisely.

Adverse effects are undesirable reactions that occur only in some patients. Usually they are unrelated to dosage and are uncommon. They can be allergic reactions such as may occur with any drug or food; for example, an itchy, red rash may develop on the arms. Some adverse reactions are more serious, even life-threatening. When an adverse reaction occurs, the drug must be stopped. After the reaction subsides, treatment may be resumed with another drug, preferably one that is chemically unrelated.

A third type of undesired effect is sometimes caused by the interference of one drug in the action or metabolism of another drug. Some examples of drug interaction are given later.

RESPONSE OF SYMPTOMS

The symptoms of Parkinson's disease are not all equally responsive to drug treatment. Some symptoms respond quite readily, others less so, and some not at all. In fact some symptoms may be exacerbated. For example, the tendency to constipation common in Parkinson patients is increased by some anti-Parkinson drugs.

Patients often ask for a drug to control one symptom and another to ease another symptom, but the drugs do not work that way. It just is not possible to treat parkinsonism symptom by symptom. In general the anti-Parkinson drugs act on the parkinsonian state as a whole, and they do not differ in their relative specificity for one or another symptom. It was once thought that some drugs were better for rigidity and others for tremor or akinesia. This line of thinking is reflected in the trade names of some drugs; for example, Akineton (biperiden) implies an action on akinesia. Treatment based on such concepts led to complicated regimens with three, four, or even five drugs being given at the same time. Fortunately these views have been largely abandoned. Side effects are more frequent with multiple drug regimens, and it is generally easier to adjust the dosage of one drug than the dosages of several. If excessive side effects or adverse effects develop, it may be difficult to judge which of several drugs is responsible and which to stop or reduce. In short it is better to use one drug well than three not so well. It also is good practice, as well as common sense, to use as few drugs as possible in the lowest doses that give a satisfactory result.

Generally, among the classic triad of symptoms, rigidity is the most responsive to drug treatment. With levodopa therapy it is usually completely abolished and often replaced by hypotonia of the muscle; that is, the disturbance of muscle tone we call rigidity is actually overcorrected! The patient whose muscles are hypotonic looks "loose jointed" in bodily movements. The anticholinergic drugs can also alleviate rigidity, but rarely to the point of hypotonia.

Tremor is greatly reduced and often abolished by drug treatment. Of course even if tremor is reduced by 80% or so, there is still some tremor and so the effect of treatment is not always fully appreciated. All the anti-Parkinson drugs relieve tremor to some extent. Sedative drugs also alleviate tremor but to a lesser extent and only at the expense of some drowsiness. Levodopa sometimes increases the tremor of Parkinson's disease at the outset of therapy, but with continued treatment it relieves the tremor more effectively than any other drug available today.

Bradykinesia, or akinesia, is reduced by all the drugs, and when mild or moderate, it is usually abolished completely. When severe, however, it may be only partially reduced. In patients with severe parkinsonism, akinesia is the most distressing persistent symptom. In these cases rigidity is abolished, and very little tremor is left, but significant akinesia may persist. Sometimes akinesia reappears briefly for a few minutes or so without tremor or rigidity.

Drug treatment can restore the automatic associated movements—eye blink, swallowing, swing of the arms during walking, expressive gestures, facial expressive movements, etc.—to normal or near normal. The amplitude of the voice and modulation of speech is improved. Disturbances of gait are also improved. The step becomes brisker, and the ability to walk slowly or rapidly and to turn around briskly can be restored. Shuffling, festination, and propulsion can be greatly diminished or completely abolished.

Feelings of numbness, weakness, aching or pulling pains, tightness, etc. are relieved. The excessive sweating and oiliness of the skin are also diminished. Pooling of saliva and drooling are greatly ameliorated. Painful cramps and the rare heat sensations called thermal paresthesias tend to be diminished but sometimes persist despite good treatment.

Because the disease continues to progress despite the best treatment possible, symptoms once well controlled may reemerge, or new symptoms may develop in the course of time. For example, a patient who had only mild tremor and rigidity on one side when the diagnosis of Parkinson's disease was made and treatment first begun may several years later experience some intermittent reappearance of the same tremor; or a new symptom may develop, such as a tendency at times to drag one foot during walking. In these circumstances patients often ask if the drug has lost its effect or if they themselves have become "resistant" to the drugs. Chances are it is merely a question of gradual progression of the disease so that the duration of response to a given dose has decreased. As a result tremor may reappear when the the last dose begins to wear off. A change in the timing of the doses through the day or a change in medication will probably control the symptoms again. Sometimes a change in activity or diet may alter the metabolism of the drugs and render a previously effective dose less effective. Levodopa is especially sensitive to changes in eating habits. Its absorption may be delayed by foods rich in protein. Thus if there has been a sudden loss of benefit from an effective drug regimen, it is a good idea to check for recent changes in diet, life style, or activity, and also to check if the change coincides with the introduction of a new drug into the patient's regimen.

Whereas some patients require increases in the dosage over the years, others develop an increased sensitivity. Usually the dosage of levodopa required, once established, remains about the same for years: After many years it may be useful to modify the schedule of doses through the day. Somewhat smaller doses taken at shorter intervals may then prove helpful—or a change to the slow-release formulation or the addition of another drug.

Rarely the drugs produce results opposite to those expected. Whereas they relieve symptoms at one dose, they may increase certain symptoms at a higher dose. This is called a "paradoxical" effect. One of our patients, when first seen, was troubled chiefly by a slowness of movement and stiffness in his legs while walking. Treatment with levodopa at the modest dose improved these symptoms to a moderate degree. However, when the dose was increased further, he failed to improve. In fact his wife reported that at a higher dose he was actually slower and stiffer. When the patient discontinued his medication for several days for a religious fast, he reported that he actually felt better. He then remained off his medication completely for several more days. Although he felt better at first, he gradually became worse again and all his original symptoms returned. He then resumed taking levodopa and found that he felt best at an intermediate dose. Puzzled by this observation, we admitted him to the hospital to study his reaction to levodopa more objectively. He was treated with a very small dose for several days, then with a full dose for several days. He was examined hourly during the day, and blood samples were taken to measure the amount of the drug. When the results were in, it was clear that he did indeed have a striking paradoxical response to levodopa treatment. The higher the dose he took and the higher the blood level, the greater were his symptoms: He was slower and walked more stiffly. When he set out to walk, his feet seemed to hesitate as if his shoes were momentarily stuck to the floor. This curious phenomenon has been called "start hesitation" and has occasionally been observed as a paradoxical effect in patients on higher doses.

Thus if a new symptom appears after an increase in the dose, the possibility of a paradoxical response should be considered. In such circumstances there may be a narrow range over which the dosage is optimal. Going above or below that range makes matters worse! Finding the optimal dose may require considerable patience and care in making dosage adjustments. It requires close cooperation of patient and doctor.

DRUG HOLIDAYS

It was first noted some years ago during the initial trials of levodopa that when therapy was withdrawn for 1 week or more and then resumed, it was more effective for a time. This observation led to the widespread use of "drug holidays" in the hope of restoring responsiveness to levodopa. However, with further experience enthusiasm for the drug holiday declined. It proved useful only in the rare instances when patients had severe involuntary movements and mental disturbances. It may be a difficult, unpleasant, and even dangerous experience for the patient, and should be done only by a physician experienced in its use, preferably in the hospital.

6

Anticholinergic Drugs

For a century before the advent of levodopa, anticholinergic drugs were the only treatment available for parkinsonism. They have been largely supplanted by levodopa and other drugs. We rarely use them in our own practice. However, they may still be helpful occasionally in patients to supplement the effects of levodopa or in the rare patients who cannot tolerate levodopa. It is also important to be aware that the anticholinergic properties of drugs given for some other reason (for example, antihistamines taken as a cold remedy) will have some effect on Parkinson's disease symptoms. Therefore we should briefly review this class of drugs.

The first anticholinergic drugs were derived from plants. Just how they came to be used in treating parkinsonism is not clear. The first definite mention of their use for this purpose seems to be a comment in a doctoral thesis dated 1869 by a medical student in Paris that Professor Charcot was then administering some hyoscine to patients with Parkinson's disease. Hyoscine, also called scopolamine, is the active ingredient of the plant *Datura stramonium,* known popularly as jimsonweed or thorn apple. Wine extracts of the plant had been used for centuries as tincture of stramonium in the treatment of stomach cramps and abdominal colic. Closely related botanical preparations are the alcoholic extract, or tincture, of the plant *Hyoscyamus niger* (black henbane) and the extract of *Atropa belladonna* (deadly nightshade). The active principles are named hyoscyamine and atropine, respectively. The plants are members of the potato family, called Solanaceae in botanical terminology. The extracts are alkaline and bitter-tasting; hence they are termed *solanaceous alkaloids.*

Tincture of belladonna and its active ingredients (or principles), atropine and hyoscine (scopolamine), are still used for some purposes in medical practice. They act on the vagus nerve, which controls the stomach, intestine, bladder, and heart. The vagus nerve transmits its influence to the various organs through the action of a chemical intermediary, or messenger. The messenger is a simple chemical substance called acetylcholine. The solanaceous alkaloids work by blocking the action of acetylcholine and thus are classed as *anticholinergic drugs.*

For some unknown reason patients with post-encephalitic parkinsonism tolerated much larger doses of anticholinergic drugs than can normal people or even patients with Parkinson's disease. The post-encephalitic cases were also quite numerous during the 1920s and 1930s, and thus particular attention was directed to their treatment. Various treatment regimens with these alkaloids were developed, such as Roemer's high-dosage atropine treatment, in which doses that today would be considered fantastic were routinely employed.

The high dosages of the drugs used produced side effects including mental confusion, mild incoordination, slurred speech, and forgetfulness, which collectively were known as the "belladonna jag." Similar symptoms of anticholinergic intoxication may occur in Parkinson's disease patients with much smaller doses. Other side effects included blurring of vision, dryness of the mouth, loss of sweating, and constipation.

SYNTHETIC ANTICHOLINERGIC DRUGS

Once the chemical structure of acetylcholine was known, chemists were able to synthesize new chemical compounds in the laboratory to imitate or block its action. Thus synthetic anticholinergic drugs were developed in the hope that they would be more effective. One of the first of these drugs, trihexyphenidyl (Artane), was introduced as an anti-Parkinson drug circa 1949–1951. It appeared to have fewer side effects than the older potato plant drugs and to be equally effective. It was rapidly followed by three other closely related drugs: procyclidine (Kemadrin), cycrimine (Pagitane), and biperiden (Akineton). Of these, only trihexyphenidyl and biperiden are still available. Trihexyphenidyl is also marketed under different names.

For most of the 20 years from 1950 to 1970 (that is, until the introduction of levodopa), trihexyphenidyl and its cousins were the chief anti-Parkinson drugs in common use. But with the advent of levodopa their use gradually declined. We rarely use these agents today in ordinary Parkinson's disease. They are more useful in treating drug-induced parkinsonism. In contrast to levodopa these drugs can reverse the parkinsonism induced by tranquilizer drugs.

Trihexyphenidyl is available in white 2- and 5-mg scored tablets and in a blue 5-mg slow-release capsule. The normal starting dose is one 2-mg tablet three times daily. For patients who are sensitive to the side effects of anticholinergic drugs, the 2-mg scored tablet may be broken in half, and 1 mg taken two or three times daily. If the 2-mg tablet is well tolerated, the dose may be increased to one 5-mg tablet three times daily. More than 15 mg daily is rarely helpful in Parkinson's disease. Indeed, most patients cannot tolerate larger doses.

Another synthetic anticholinergic agent widely used in treating parkinsonism is benztropine mesylate (Cogentin). The molecular structure of this drug is closely patterned after that of atropine; hence the "tropine" in its generic name. It is somewhat more potent than trihexyphenidyl and is consequently made in smaller dosage forms: 0.5-, 1- and 2-mg tablets. It is also available, as is biperiden (Akineton), in a liquid form for injection with a hypodermic needle. It is used to treat parkinsonism and other similar reactions to tranquilizer drugs. A single injection can terminate the tranquilizer reaction within minutes.

ANTIHISTAMINES

Atropine was once widely used in the treatment of asthma. The search for a drug that would have atropine's effect in asthma and other allergies but not its anticholinergic effects led to the development of the drug diphenhydramine (Benadryl). Introduced around 1946, it proved highly successful and was soon widely used in the treatment of hay fever, asthma and many other allergies. Its success led to the introduction of many related drugs for the treatment of allergies. Their beneficial effect is thought to be due to their ability to block the action of the natural substance *histamine* formed in the body during allergic reactions; these drugs are thus classified as *antihistamines*. Some of these, notably diphenhydramine, were accidentally found to have some effect on the symptoms of Parkinson's disease. Although diphenhydramine itself has not been marketed and advertised to physicians as an anti-Parkinson drug, it has nonetheless been widely used in treating parkinsonism. The dosage required to affect parkinsonian symptoms is 50 mg two to four times daily.

Many other antihistamines not normally thought of as anti-Parkinson drugs nevertheless affect parkinsonian symptoms. The reason antihistamines may be helpful in parkinsonism has nothing to do with their properties as antihistamines; instead it is the fact that all have some anticholinergic properties. Trihexyphenidyl is approximately 25 times more potent an anticholinergic agent than is diphenhydramine, and so the latter is used in dosages 25 times as great. Thus 50 mg of diphenhydramine is as effective in relieving parkinsonian symptoms as 2 mg of trihexyphenidyl. Any drug having some anticholinergic effect also has some anti-Parkinson effect.

CHOLINERGIC DRUGS

There are drugs that enhance or imitate the action in the nervous system of the chemical messenger acetylcholine. Naturally these are called *cholinergic drugs*. It is an interesting fact that cholinergic drugs exacerbate the symptoms of parkinsonism! For example, injection of a small dose of the drug physostigmine (Antilirium), which enhances the action of acetylcholine in the brain, produces within minutes a marked increase in the tremor, rigidity, and other symptoms of parkinsonism. This effect subsides spontaneously within about 45 minutes.

It is clearly a good idea for Parkinson patients to avoid cholinergic drugs. In practice, however, very few cholinergic drugs are used, and the likelihood of a patient encountering one inadvertently (that is, one that can get into the brain and exacerbate parkinsonian symptoms) is quite remote. Only two cholinergic drugs are used at all extensively in medical practice: pilocarpine, used in the form of eyedrops to treat glaucoma; and bethanechol (Urecholine), used to stimulate the bladder. These drugs do not affect parkinsonian symptoms. The manufacturer of bethanechol lists parkinsonism in the prescribing directions as a condition in which this drug should not be used. However, we have often used it to stimulate sluggish bladders of Parkinson patients and have never seen an adverse effect on the parkinsonian symptoms. It is highly unlikely that bethanechol in the doses ordinarily used will have an effect on the Parkinson state. Recently several new cholinergic drugs—for example, tacrine (Cognex)—have been introduced as treatment for Alzheimer's disease. They may partially correct the forgetfulness that is a common symptom of that condition. These drugs should not be given to Parkinson patients.

ANTICHOLINERGIC DRUG INTOXICATION

All the drugs discussed in this chapter depend on their anticholinergic properties for their usefulness in treating parkinsonism; that is, they block the action of the chemical messenger acetylcholine in the brain. By the same token their side effects are due to the same mechanism. Blocking acetylcholine too severely produces undesirable effects, and the side effects are essentially the same with all of the anticholinergic drugs. There is a common pattern that we term "anticholinergic intoxication."

The most common side effects are dryness of the mouth, blurring of near vision, constipation, and weakening of the bladder. In addition there is a whole range of mental side effects. Dryness of the mouth is due to a reduced flow of saliva. The saliva is also thicker and harder to swallow. The throat and nose may feel dry. The symptom is most marked when first starting treatment with anticholinergics. Partial tolerance develops within a few weeks, and most patients find it only a minor nuisance with continuing treatment. Some seek relief by sucking on bitter lemon candies or other hard sweets.

Blurring of near vision is due to the fact that anticholinergic drugs tend to diminish the action of the fine muscle in the eye that changes the shape of the lens to focus on near objects. Normally the eye has universal focus for everything more than 18 inches away. To get a sharp view of objects at closer range, it is necessary to change the shape of the lens of the eye. This change is called "accommodation." Ophthalmologists regularly put drops of atropine or a synthetic anticholinergic in the eye for the purpose of "paralyzing accommodation," so that the optical properties of the eye can be tested precisely. Taking an anticholinergic drug by mouth produces the same effect, but to a lesser degree. For this reason many patients notice difficulty in reading or doing close work when they first start on anticholinergic drugs. People normally have increasing difficulty with near vision after reaching middle age, called presbyopia. Age renders the individual more susceptible to this effect of anticholinergics. In addition anticholinergics cause the pupil to open a bit more widely. This may also contribute to the blurring of near vision. Generally the visual effect of the anticholinergics diminishes after a while. If it proves persistent, however, a new set of reading glasses can be obtained.

The tendency to widen or dilate the pupil may exacerbate glaucoma. Patients who have Parkinson's disease and glaucoma should be carefully checked by their eye doctor when treatment with anticholinergics is begun. If the glaucoma is under proper treatment or has been surgically corrected, there is usually no difficulty. The eye doctor can readily check the pressure of the eye to make sure that the treatment for the parkinsonism does not adversely affect the glaucoma.

Anticholinergic drugs typically slow the motor activity of the intestine. The waves of contraction called peristalsis are slowed. It is for this reason that many anticholinergic drugs are employed for the treatment of disorders of the stomach and intestine; for example, the drug diphenoxylate/atropine sulfate (Lomotil) is commonly used to treat diarrhea. However, by the same token the constipation of Parkinson's disease may be somewhat increased. This is rarely a serious problem, but if constipation is troublesome, it can be managed with gentle laxatives.

A similar calming effect is exerted by anticholinergic drugs on the musculature of the urinary bladder. In a sense these drugs sedate the bladder. This may be helpful to the patient troubled with urinary urgency who needs to get up several times during the night to void. An anticholinergic drug given at bedtime may help relieve this symptom. Indeed the drug hyoscyamine (Cystospaz), one of the solanaceous alkaloids mentioned earlier, is commonly prescribed by urologists to control this symptom; another is oxybutynin chloride (Ditropan), a synthetic anticholinergic. However, in the older male patient who has trouble due to an enlarged prostate gland obstructing the flow of urine, this calming effect can lead to urinary retention. Thus anticholinergic drugs are given with caution to patients who have symptoms of prostatic obstruction. The need to pass a catheter can usually be averted by using very small doses of the drug. It may of course be necessary to operate on the prostate. A specialist in urology should be consulted before symptoms of urinary obstruction reach a severe stage.

The mental effects of anticholinergic drugs are important and, in many ways, very interesting. The fact that ingestion of the leaves of jimsonweed, henbane, or deadly nightshade can cause mental disturbances has been known since ancient times. Abuse of these botanicals for psychedelic effects has been described repeatedly. Nearly every year one sees news reports of children becoming delirious after eating jimsonweed leaves. The symptoms include confusion, agitation, hallucinations, stupor, and in severe intoxication, coma. The symptoms subside within a day or two except for amnesia for the episode.

The first and most common mental side effect noticeable in patients being treated with any anticholinergic drug is forgetfulness, mainly for recent events. Patients may forget where they left their glasses a minute ago or what they went to buy at the corner store. Occasionally mild confusion then appears. Visual illusions are especially frequent. Familiar objects may be mistaken for something else. The patient may mention seeing worms on the floor, misinterpreting a pattern design in the flooring because it seems to move. Spectral illusions generally of a benign if not pleasing character are experienced. There may be hallucinations of people or animals roaming about the house. Most commonly there seem to be complex scenes with a group of people wandering about, having a party. They may be smaller than normal and seem to go about their business without disturbing the patient. Patients may experience these visions for long periods of time but are afraid to mention them to anyone for fear of being thought "crazy." Finally, however, in a moment of confusion, the patient reacts to these illusions. Some patients angrily order the strangers out of the house, accuse them of stealing, or call the police to chase them away. At this point the patient's family, not having previously noticed anything out of the ordinary, become alarmed. There is, however, no reason to be frightened. These disturbances disappear if the dosage of the anticholinergic drug is reduced. The physician should check to see if these disturbances followed a change in medication or the addition of a new drug. A patient who has been doing well on a standard dose of, say, trihexyphenidyl may suddenly develop such mental disturbances when another drug is added. For example, the patient may have taken an antihistamine because of hay fever symptoms. The anticholinergic properties of the antihistamine added to the anticholinergic properties of trihexyphenidyl then carried the patient over the threshold into a mild state of anticholinergic intoxication. Usually the disturbance subsides within a day or so after the new drug is discontinued. If there has been no change of medication, the patient's drug regimen may be revised downward. Usually it is not a good idea to give a tranquilizer unless there is severe agitation. Many of the commonly used major tranquilizers also have some anticholinergic properties, and so the confusion and hallucinations may be increased even if the agitation is controlled for a few hours.

Some patients are very sensitive to the toxic mental effects of the anticholinergic drugs and cannot tolerate any of these drugs, not even very mild ones such as the antihistamines. A few patients develop these mental reactions even after the mildest sleep medications. Rarely a patient experiences these disturbances spontaneously, on no treatment at all. There is probably something inherent to Parkinson's disease that makes one susceptible to these mental disturbances.

Another effect of the anticholinergic drugs that may be good or bad, depending on the circumstances, is the tendency to reduce sweating. Excessive sweating, sometimes occurring irregularly in bursts, is an occasional symptom of Parkinson's disease. Anticholinergic drugs can diminish this excessive perspiration— sometimes not as much as desired and sometimes too much. We depend on sweating to cool our bodies in warm weather. The brain controls the amount of sweat we produce, thereby regulating body temperature. Anticholinergic drugs may impair this regulation, and in warm weather fever and even coma may result. This is a rare occurrence today but was a familiar problem years ago when large doses of atropine were commonly used in treating parkinsonism.

ADVERSE REACTIONS

Adverse reactions have been very rare with the anticholinergic drugs. We have never seen one, but there are reports in medical journals of isolated instances of allergic skin rashes, inflammation of the liver, and a rare toxic effect on the bone marrow resulting in a lack of white blood corpuscles.

AMANTADINE (SYMMETREL)

A Parkinson's disease patient of the late Dr. Robert Schwab reported that while taking the drug amantadine (Symmetrel) as protection against catching the flu she felt better. This drug had been developed as an antiviral agent and is protective against the flu virus. Dr. Schwab confirmed this observation and then treated other Parkinson patients with amantadine, finding that many of these patients looked and felt better while taking the drug. Other doctors also tried amantadine in their Parkinson patients and corroborated Dr. Schwab's report.

Amantadine does indeed possess some property that partially alleviates the symptoms of Parkinson's disease. Its side effects—blurring of vision, constipation, mental confusion, dryness of the mouth—suggest that it acts as an anticholinergic drug. However, laboratory studies failed to show a direct acetylcholine blocking effect. It had been reported that amantadine enhances the function of dopamine nerve cells, and it was thought that it mimicked the effects of L-dopa, the precursor of dopamine. However, this effect has only been shown in test tube experiments, with amounts of the drug far greater than the dosages that can be used in humans. Thus although it is still often referred to as a "dopaminergic" drug, we do not agree that amantadine can be so classified. More recently scien-

FIG. 8. Livido reticularis is the purplish mottling of the skin on the leg of a patient treated with amantadine.

tists have found that it indirectly blocks the action of acetylcholine. Thus we consider amantadine to be a novel type of anticholinergic agent.

Amantadine is available in a 100-mg red capsule. The normal dose is one capsule two or three times daily, although some patients may take as many as four. It is also available in a liquid solution. Since it may augment the side effects of anticholinergic drugs such as trihexyphenidyl, care is usually taken to change doses slowly when the two drugs are used simultaneously. We rarely use both drugs together.

A unique and unusual side effect of amantadine is the appearance of a curious faint purplish mottling of the skin of the legs and sometimes the arms due to blood pooling in small veins in the skin. It usually appears only after several months and may take 1 to 2 months to subside after the drug is stopped. This unusual side effect is apparently harmless. It is called *livido reticularis* (Fig. 8). Sometimes the purplish mottling is accompanied by swelling of the feet and ankles due to the accumulation of water in the soft tissues. The medical term for this accumulation of water is *edema*. Although it may be ungainly and worrisome, this too appears to be harmless and disappears when amantadine is discontinued.

Another curious property of amantadine is that it may lose its effectiveness after several months. However, if the patient stops taking the drug for a while and then uses it again, it usually regains its effectiveness. Although this phenomenon occurs in only some patients, it is still worthwhile to determine whether amantadine is still effective when a patient has been taking it for some time. We often advise our patients in such circumstances to discontinue the drug for a week or so. If there is no change and the patient does not feel worse, there seems no point in taking it again. It may then be discontinued completely and tried again after a month or two. On the other hand, if the patient is definitely worse after stopping the amantadine, drug treatment should be promptly resumed because it is clear that the drug is worth taking.

7

From L-Dopa to Levodopa

. . . what drug can make a withered palsy cease to shake?
The Two Voices—Alfred Tennyson

L-Dopa is the most effective substance currently available for the treatment of Parkinson's disease. Its full chemical name is L-3,4-dihydroxyphenylalanine. Chemists have for many years abbreviated this cumbersome name to the simpler "dopa" or "L-dopa." Persons not versed in the language of chemistry sometimes fear that the name dopa has a more sinister meaning. Patients often ask if the drug L-dopa contains "dope." Many wonder if it is a Spanish drug, for they understand L-dopa to be El Dopa. Others inquire about the ingredients of L-dopa.

L-dopa is in fact merely a simple chemical substance occurring in nature in both animals and plants. It is not a mixture of ingredients but a single rather simple molecule belonging to a class of substances known to chemists as amino acids and composed of atoms of carbon, hydrogen, oxygen, and nitrogen. The arrangement of these atoms in the dopa molecule is shown in Fig. 9. Its shape in three-dimensional space is such that the dopa molecule can exist in two forms, each the mirror image of the other, just as the right hand is the mirror image of the left. The bones and ligaments of both hands are connected in exactly the same way, yet the two hands are not exactly the same in three-dimensional space; they cannot fit in the same glove. The two forms of the dopa molecule are designated the levo form (from the Latin *laevo*, meaning left) and the dextro form (from the Latin prefix *dexter*, meaning right)—or more simply, the L- and D-forms.

Many molecules exist in duplicate mirror forms, such as L-glucose and D-glucose, L-amphetamine and D-amphetamine, L-tryptophan and D-tryptophan, and so on. Just as your right hand cannot fit in a left-hand glove, so the L-forms of these molecules cannot fit in the same spaces as the D-forms. Consequently the two forms of these molecules often have different physical properties, form crystals of different shapes, and behave differently in the biological world. It is a remarkable fact that plants and animals make and use only the L-forms! Only the L-form of dopa is found in nature, and only the L-form is effective in treating Parkinson's disease. The D-form is inert!

FIG. 9. Model of the dopa molecule. The nitrogen and its attached hydrogen atom form an amine group, which confers the chemical properties of an alkali on the molecule. The group at the far right end of the molecule—consisting of a carbon atom holding an oxygen atom with two arms (or bonds) and an oxygen-hydrogen combination with one bond—is called a carboxyl group. This confers the properties of an acid on the molecule. Dopa is thus an amino acid. Removal of the carboxyl group—a step called decarboxylation and controlled by an enzyme aptly enough called a decarboxylase—converts the dopa molecule to a dopamine molecule.

L-dopa was first discovered in 1908 in the broad bean or fava bean (*Vicia faba*) used in Mediterranean cooking. It is also present in the velvet bean (*Mucuna pruriens*), the locoweed, and certain other related legumes. Botanists have suggested that L-dopa serves to protect the plants from insects.

L-dopa also occurs in the animal kingdom, where it plays an important role as an intermediate substance in the metabolism of adrenaline, the hormone secreted into the circulation by the adrenal gland to prepare the body for "fight or flight" in an emergency. The adrenal gland makes adrenaline in a series of chemical reactions that begin with the amino acid tyrosine, an ingredient of our diet. Tyrosine is found mainly in the proteins we eat every day. An ordinary American hamburger, for example, contains 1 to 2 grams of tyrosine. When we eat a hamburger or other meat, the protein molecules in it are broken down during digestion to simpler molecules called peptides. These in turn are further broken down into their component amino acids. After being absorbed by the intestines, the amino acids are transported in the blood first to the liver and then to other organs throughout the body. Most of the tyrosine we absorb from our daily diet is used to build new protein. A very small proportion is taken up from the circulation by the cells of the adrenal gland. There it is immediately converted by a single molecular re-arrangement to L-dopa. L-dopa in turn is promptly changed into dopamine via an-other chemical reaction. In turn dopamine is changed into norepinephrine, and in the final step in this metabolic pathway noradrenaline is converted into adrena-line. The adrenaline is then stored by the cells of the adrenal gland in little pack-ets, which can be seen under the electron microscope, until such time as the gland receives a signal from the nervous system to release it into the blood stream.

This pathway of sequential chemical reactions occurs in exactly the same way in the substantia nigra of the brain. Here, however, the process ends with the for-mation of dopamine. The dopamine is then stored in these cells and their fibers, which spread throughout the corpus striatum, until released to function as a chemical messenger to other nerve cells. In other areas of the nervous system (for example, in the sympathetic nerves), the process ends with the formation of noradrenaline.

The step from tyrosine to dopa in the adrenal gland and the brain is strictly con-trolled and is called a "rate-limiting" step. Feeding large amounts of tyrosine does not result in the formation of larger amounts of dopamine or of noradrenaline or adrenaline. This is not surprising. If it were not so, every time we ate a lot of pro-tein we would have too much adrenaline in our systems. However, the step from L-dopa to dopamine is not subject to such control, and so it is possible to increase the amount of dopamine formed in the brain by feeding large amounts of L-dopa. Thus tyrosine has little effect in treating parkinsonism, whereas L-dopa is very ef-fective. Essentially L-dopa relieves the symptoms of parkinsonism by restoring brain dopamine at least partially to normal levels. L-Dopa itself is inert. All of its actions are due to the dopamine derived from it in the various organs of the body.

LEVODOPA TREATMENT

L-Dopa is the name employed by chemists to describe this interesting substance. However, L-dopa prepared for use as a drug is officially termed levodopa. This is the international generic name of the medicinal form of L-dopa. It is marketed, of course, under various trade names by different pharmaceutical firms.

Levodopa taken by mouth passes through the stomach into the duodenum and then to the upper and small intestine where it is absorbed. The process of ab-sorption takes place over a period of several hours. We can study this process by measuring (via chemical means) the amount of levodopa in the blood at various intervals after a dose is ingested. Measurements done on different patients or on the same patient on different days vary somewhat, but in general the level of lev-odopa in the blood (normally zero) gradually rises to a peak value approximate-ly 30 minutes to 2 hours after a dose is taken by mouth, then gradually falls back to zero again within 4 to 6 hours. The results of such a study, plotted as a graph, are seen in Fig. 10.

From such studies a number of things have been found to influence the absorption of levodopa. One of the most important is the amount and type of food in the stomach. Solid food, especially food containing protein, delays the absorption of levodopa and may reduce the amount taken up in the circulation. Many patients are aware of this effect of food. They have observed that the relief of their symptoms is greater and comes on more rapidly when they take a dose of levodopa on an empty stomach than when they take it after a meal. Many have also noted that their usual dose may have little or no effect if taken after a hearty steak dinner. Patients on a low-protein diet need less levodopa to obtain the same result they experience with higher doses on a regular diet.

If the stomach is excessively acid, it empties into the duodenum more slowly, and consequently the absorption of levodopa is delayed. In such circumstances taking some milk or an antacid tablet with the levodopa improves the absorption of levodopa. Some patients report that chewing the levodopa tablet rather than

FIG. 10. Graph shows the amount of levodopa at various times in the blood of a patient after a single dose was administered at 9:00 A.M. Blood was then drawn from a vein each hour until 4:00 P.M. The highest blood level of levodopa was measured in the sample taken at 12:00 noon.

swallowing it provides faster relief of their symptoms. They use this trick for a "booster" effect, usually with supplementary midafternoon doses. Levodopa, however, is not absorbed from the mouth.

Once absorbed into the circulation, levodopa travels throughout the entire body. A large proportion of the dose taken by mouth ends up in muscles, fat stores, the liver, skin, kidney, and other organs. Most of it is rapidly converted to dopamine in the blood vessels in the various organs, especially the kidney, and is excreted in the urine in the form of various inactive substances.

Only a very small proportion of the oral dose of levodopa, probably less than 1%, ultimately penetrates the brain. There it is selectively taken up by the dopamine nerve cells of the substantia nigra and possibly also by other cells and then converted to dopamine. In this manner the brain stores of dopamine may be at least partially replenished.

Of course some time is required for the levodopa to leave the bloodstream, cross the walls of the blood vessels, enter the brain, and reach the dopamine cells, where it may then be converted to dopamine. Animal studies indicate that this delay is usually 15 to 30 minutes. Thus if the peak blood level of levodopa is reached 1 hour after ingestion, the peak brain level of dopamine must be reached approximately 1 hour and 15 minutes to 1 hour and 30 minutes after ingestion. Of course some effects may begin to be felt 20 to 30 minutes after taking a dose of levodopa by mouth, but the full effect does not occur until at least an hour and a half later. The newly formed dopamine in the brain joins the dopamine formed in the normal manner from tyrosine as just described. In this way brain dopamine stores are replenished, and the symptoms of parkinsonism are correspondingly diminished.

Levodopa treatment, however, is not a cure. So far as we know, it does not affect the basic disease process—whatever it may be—responsible for the dysfunction of the brain's dopamine cells or bring back those that may have deteriorated. It merely helps the dopamine nerve cells make dopamine more readily. Apparently it helps the cells function better despite their illness. Levodopa treatment is thus a symptomatic treatment. That is, it is a treatment that can relieve symptoms without correcting the underlying or primary cause. It may also be considered a replacement therapy—that is, a treatment based on replacing a substance essential to the body's economy that is deficient. The same may be said of other forms of treatment in modern medicine: thyroid hormone treatment for hypothyroidism, for example, or insulin treatment for diabetes. In diabetes mellitus there is a deficiency of insulin, the hormone that regulates sugar metabolism throughout the body. The diabetic patient may be given insulin by injection to provide the body with the insulin it needs but is unable to make itself in sufficient amounts. In this way the disturbance in sugar metabolism that causes so much of the trouble in diabetes can be corrected. However, insulin does not cure diabetes. It does not correct the basic disease—whatever it is—and restore the body's ability to make proper amounts of insulin.

When levodopa treatment is first begun, the patient feels a gradual improvement over a period of several days. An appreciable response is usually achieved within 3 to 5 days, but still further improvement builds up more slowly over the subsequent weeks. The full effect of treatment may not be apparent for 2 to 3 months of continuing treatment. Most patients are not aware of the effect of each individual dose. Nor are they aware of any definite change if they miss a given dose. If a dose is missed inadvertently, there is little point in trying to make up the lost dose by taking more pills the next time the medicine is due. When treatment is stopped for any reason, the parkinsonian symptoms return gradually over a period of several days. Little change may be noted the first day. Definite change is experienced the second day after stopping treatment and still more the third and fourth days. Most of the benefit of levodopa treatment is lost by the fourth or fifth days, but it may take 1 to 2 weeks before the effect of levodopa is completely gone. The slowness of the response to treatment and the long duration of the response when treatment is stopped indicate that in most patients the brain is able to store dopamine for some period of time, and that to fill up the dopamine stores may require several months of continuing treatment. It is as if a large reservoir is being filled through a small opening with a small bucket. Many buckets and some time are required to fill the reservoir to its full capacity.

MOTOR FLUCTUATIONS

Some patients after a period of years of treatment feel the effect of each dose of levodopa. They can tell when a given dose begins to work, to diminish their symptoms. They can also tell when the effect of a given dose wears off. Such patients may also experience some return of their parkinsonian symptoms in the morning, before the first dose of the day. They seem to have lost the "sleep benefit" that most patients receive. Apparently the levodopa effect wears off overnight presumably because the dopamine reserves diminished during the long interval between the last dose at night and the first dose the following morning. In other words these patients do not have a sufficiently long enough response to levodopa to maintain full control of their symptoms for a long time. They are said to have primarily a short-duration response, which may reflect a decreased capacity to store dopamine. The reservoir is leaky, or it has become smaller.

Patients who note that the effectiveness of each dose begins to wear off after 3 to 4 hours or more may benefit from newer controlled-release preparations of levodopa (Sinemet CR or Madopar HBS). These formulations contain the same ingredients as standard tablets but are designed to release levodopa more slowly. They therefore provide steadier concentrations of dopamine to the basal ganglia over a longer time period, and their effectiveness does not depend on the ability of the brain to store dopamine. Patients with mild or moderate fluctuations taking controlled-release levodopa usually experience fewer wearing-off symptoms and can often take fewer doses each day.

In a small percentage of patients the response to levodopa appears to be chiefly of the short-duration variety. These patients fluctuate markedly from a state of parkinsonism to a state of normal movement and back again several times a day. The change from one state to the other may take place quite rapidly. Some patients have said that it felt as if an electric switch had been turned on or off. For this reason this phenomenon has been termed the *on–off* effect. The fluctuations can be smoothed out to some extent by adjusting the dosage schedule to the duration of the individual patient's response. Thus instead of taking levodopa only three or four times daily as is usual, such a patient might take it every 3 hours— or even every 2 hours—through the day. It is rarely worthwhile to take levodopa more frequently than every 2 hours. The precise timing can be very important and must be carefully worked out, by trial and error, in each patient. Generally results are best if the patient follows a definite schedule strictly "by the clock" and works closely with the doctor to develop the most appropriate schedule. Some patients with this on–off problem are able to judge sufficiently in advance when an "off" phase is coming and so take their levodopa dose when they feel the need. However, in our experience, most patients who self-regulate their dosage schedules depending on their own subjective feeling do poorly. They tend to overdose themselves and become confused about how much to take and when to take it. Often they cannot tell whether their symptoms at any one time are due to overdosage or underdosage, and fail to distinguish the symptoms of parkinsonism from the side effects of levodopa.

NAUSEA AND VOMITING

Dopamine formed from taking the medication levodopa accumulates not only in the corpus striatum but in other brain areas as well. This may be all to the good, but it may also give rise to undesired side effects. A major side effect when levodopa therapy was first being developed was nausea and vomiting. We have since learned to lessen this side effect, and it is no longer the problem it was. Moreover, levodopa is now usually given in combination with an enzyme-inhibitor drug, either carbidopa or benserazide, that prevents the conversion of levodopa to dopamine throughout the body *except* in the brain. A major benefit of this combination treatment is a marked decrease in the frequency and severity of nausea and vomiting. Nevertheless, since nausea and vomiting still occasionally occur even with the combination treatment, we should consider in some detail the mechanism of this unpleasant side effect and the methods of dealing with it that proved useful when only levodopa was available. We will discuss this again in the section on enzyme-inhibitor drugs.

There is a specialized area known as the area postrema, located in the brainstem near the junction of the brain and the spinal cord (see Fig. 2 in Chapter 1). This is the vomiting center. It contains nerve cells whose task it is to detect toxins or poisons in the circulation and to prevent further absorption of such substances by provoking the stomach to empty its contents to throw out the offending material.

The vomiting center is sensitive to levodopa, adrenaline, and many other substances. Apparently it regards levodopa, an unusual substance to find in the circulation, as an offensive material to be thrown out. As the blood level of levodopa rises approximately 30 minutes after a dose, the vomiting center may be activated. It can also be activated when levodopa is given by direct injection into the bloodstream through a vein. The vomiting induced by levodopa is not due to irritation of the stomach itself, but this makes little practical difference to the patient who experiences it. First there is a general discomfort, a sense of weakness, and a disinterest in eating. If activation of the center is more marked, there is a metallic taste in the mouth, nausea, and dizziness. These symptoms may subside after a half hour or so, especially if the patient lies down. If the activation is sufficient, vomiting occurs even if there is nothing in the stomach. The vomiting usually comes very suddenly and is very quickly over, and the patient usually feels better soon afterward.

Unfortunately the dose of levodopa required to relieve the symptoms of parkinsonism is more than enough to activate the vomiting center in most persons. There are exceptions, of course. We have seen patients who took full doses of levodopa alone from the first day of treatment and never felt any nausea. At the other extreme there are patients who never tolerate full doses of levodopa and fail to develop tolerance even after many months. In the early experiments with levodopa, this state of affairs was a major obstacle to the development of an effective means of using levodopa to treat parkinsonism. However, two facts about the vomiting center make it possible to overcome this problem in most patients.

The first of these is that repeated exposure to levodopa causes the vomiting center to gradually become accustomed to its presence and the center no longer responds to it. The second is that the vomiting center is most likely to react when the blood level of dopa is rising rapidly, that is, when the levodopa taken by mouth is absorbed especially well. Thus it is possible to "tame" the vomiting center by starting treatment with small doses of levodopa and by taking levodopa only after meals to slow its absorption. In practice the major problem has been with breakfast. Many people do not eat much for breakfast—a glass of orange juice, a cup of coffee, and toast. That is not enough to slow the absorption of levodopa. In fact the caffeine in coffee may help levodopa activate the vomiting center.

Patients taking their first doses of levodopa after such a small breakfast—or nonbreakfast, if you will—are especially apt to feel at least some nausea or loss of interest in food. As lunch time rolls around a few hours later, they may still be disinclined to eat and thus content themselves with a cup of coffee for lunch. This time, the vomiting center, still disturbed by the morning dose of levodopa, may react more violently and vomiting results. In the days before the current formulations of levodopa were available, the answers to this problem were threefold: (1) make sure that breakfast includes some solid food, preferably food containing protein; (2) change to decaffeinated coffee or tea; and (3) if necessary, reduce the morning dose of levodopa. If the patient still reacted with nausea and vomiting after trying these measures, some antivomiting drug was tried. Unfortunately the most effective antivomiting drugs antagonize levodopa. They not only block the activation of the vomiting center by levodopa but also prevent the relief of parkinsonism. So treatment had to rely on milder antivomiting drugs, and these often did the trick. They included diphenidol (Vontrol) and trimethobenzamide (Tigan). The old anti-Parkinson drugs such as trihexyphenidyl (Artane) and even the common antihistamine diphenhydramine hydrochloride (Benadryl) also give some protection against the activation of the vomiting center. Thus when beginning levodopa treatment, a patient already taking trihexyphenidyl or a drug of that class was continued on it during the initial period of levodopa treatment.

The more slowly the dose of levodopa is raised, the less likely it is that nausea and vomiting will occur. Normally it seems to take 3 to 6 months to develop full tolerance to the action of levodopa on the vomiting center. Thus the patient should not be in too great a hurry to enjoy the good effects of levodopa in full measure. Both patient and physician should be willing to wait a few months before reaching the ultimate dosage schedule. Of course personal tolerance levels vary considerably. Some patients never experience even the slightest nausea, whereas others are unable to develop a sufficient tolerance to reach effective doses of levodopa even after several years.

INVOLUNTARY MOVEMENTS

The most common side effect of levodopa treatment is the production of various involuntary movements. These include twitches, jerks, nods, gestures, twisting or writhing movements, or simple restlessness. The neurological term for these movements is *dyskinesia*. These movements can be so minimal as to be barely perceptible. When they are somewhat more obvious but still very mild, they seem to be no more than restlessness or fidgetiness. Usually patients are not aware of them until they become at least mild in magnitude. Patients usually do not mind the movements even when they are quite obvious. When severe, they become tiring and cause clumsiness and awkwardness. The rapid dance-like movements are called *chorea*. Slow, twisting movements, sustained postures, and muscle cramps are called *dystonia*. The most common movements appear at higher doses of levodopa and usually occur only for a brief period, 1 to 2 hours after the last daily dose, a time when the brain levels of dopamine are highest. This is called "peakdose" dyskinesia.

The movements can be abolished by drugs that block the action of dopamine (for example, the major tranquilizers). However, these drugs also block the desired effects of levodopa and thus are helpful only in rare emergency situations to treat overdosage with levodopa. Many treatments have been tried in the hope of finding a way of preventing the movements without also preventing the relief of parkinsonian symptoms. Thus far no entirely effective means of doing this has been found. Switching from standard levodopa to a controlled-release preparation may help to some extent because the longer-acting formulations are also designed to produce lower peak concentrations of brain dopamine. In many patients, however, the only way of handling the problem is to lower the dosage of levodopa. Unfortunately many patients then have some recurrence of their parkinsonism. Most patients prefer a compromise in which some movements are present and better relief of the parkinsonism is obtained. This dilemma is the major shortcoming of levodopa therapy.

In many ways chorea and parkinsonism are opposites. In chorea there is excessive bodily movement, whereas in parkinsonism there is too little bodily movement. In chorea the muscles are loose and floppy; in parkinsonism they are stiff and rigid. Drugs that cause parkinsonism are useful in treating chorea. The converse, it seems, is also true: Levodopa, a drug that can cause chorea, is useful in treating parkinsonism. Thus the production of chorea-like movements in a Parkinson patient reflects an overcorrection of the parkinsonism and an excessive amount of dopamine in the brain at the precise moment the movements are present. A half hour later, when the movements cease, the brain dopamine level can be presumed to have decreased to a more desirable range.

Frankly the involuntary movements are a normal, though undesirable, effect of levodopa in Parkinson patients that merely reflects the dosage. Curiously levodopa does not induce these involuntary movements so readily in patients with other disorders or in normal volunteers. Parkinsonian patients are more susceptible than other people to the chorea-inducing effect of levodopa. Other drugs that alleviate parkinsonism can also induce involuntary movements, although to a lesser extent. Of course these other drugs are also less effective in relieving the symptoms of parkinsonism. It seems then that the involuntary movements are due not only to the drug but also to something at work in the brain of Parkinson's disease patients. Just what that something may be is not known. It seems reasonable to suspect that certain changes in the brain that occur to compensate for the long-standing depletion of dopamine may be responsible.

The brain is somehow able to compensate for a great loss of dopamine for a very long time. How does it do this? One way seems to be to increase the rate at which dopamine is formed, perhaps to correct for the decreased capacity to store it. Another way the brain may compensate seems to be to increase its sensitivity to the actions of dopamine so that a smaller amount may provoke the same response. The brain cells that normally receive and respond to dopamine may thus become supersensitive to it and adapt to the diminished amount of their chemical messenger. Then when dopamine becomes available again in normal amounts (when the patient starts taking levodopa), these cells respond in an exaggerated manner. It also seems probable that other nerve cells that do not normally process levodopa can assume this function. They can convert it to dopamine, but they may release it inappropriately at the wrong times in response to the wrong signals and deliver it to unusual places. These adaptations do not seem to be reversed when levodopa therapy is begun. The involuntary movements do not diminish over time with continued treatment. No tolerance to this side effect appears to develop.

MENTAL EFFECTS OF LEVODOPA

Many patients describe a feeling of being more alert after first starting levodopa treatment. They appear more attentive and more spontaneous in their activity. They become more talkative, and they seem to have more initiative and to take more interest in the world around them. Some also complain of a feeling of nervousness, of an inner restlessness, or even "jitteriness." They may also have trouble sleeping at night. These effects are somewhat reminiscent of the effects of amphetamine and related drugs often given to combat drowsiness. This is not surprising because amphetamine works in the brain by activating the normal dopamine cells. Essentially amphetamine causes these cells to release more dopamine than they normally would in the course of their usual traffic with other nerve cells. The actions of amphetamine can be blocked by drugs that block the action of dopamine. Usually the nervousness, restlessness, and insomnia subside after a few weeks of continuing treatment. If necessary, they can be controlled with minor tranquilizing drugs.

Another similar activating effect occasionally experienced by patients is vivid dreaming. They may not have dreamed in years, but after starting levodopa treatment they again enjoy dreaming. Usually this is pleasant, but excessively vivid dreams may be distressing; rarely they amount to nightmares. The simplest way of dealing with this problem is to avoid taking a bedtime dose of levodopa or to make the bedtime dose somewhat smaller. This effect also tends to diminish in time with continued treatment.

It is often difficult to tell whether a change in behavior after starting levodopa treatment is an improvement or a side effect. The patient who finds he or she has more energy and can resume doing many things around the house that had been turned over to others is improved. However, the spouse and family may complain that the patient is too "bossy," "stubborn," or "demanding." In some cases it seems that the family resents the patient reasserting a former dominance, whereas at other times it is clear that a personality change has indeed occurred.

Increased sexual interest and activity have been described as a side effect. The increased interest is evident in a number of patients. In most it has been a partial recovery toward normal, although in some cases the increased sexual activity seemed excessive and inappropriate. Most patients, however, experience no change in libido. Some years ago the alleged effect of levodopa on sexual life attracted the interest of the press. Many of my patients who read the newspaper reports humorously asked what had been left out of their pills!

Rarely levodopa seems to induce a hyperactive behavior in which the affected patient becomes agitated or "nervous," attempts too many projects, writes numerous letters, calls everyone he knows on the telephone, and plans ambitious undertakings. This manic or hypomanic behavior may occur episodically.

It is also rare for levodopa to provoke episodes of confused, irrational behavior. These may include visual hallucinations similar to those produced by the anticholinergic drugs. However, levodopa is much less prone to produce such effects than any of the other anti-Parkinson drugs. Patients who are especially sensitive to the hallucinogenic effect of these drugs should avoid all drugs, including sleep medications, antihistamines, cough suppressants, etc., except levodopa. Even then the levodopa dosage should be adjusted very cautiously.

Levodopa can provoke a nervous breakdown in certain susceptible persons, primarily those who have had nervous breakdowns in the past or who are latent or inactive schizophrenics. Levodopa can reactivate latent schizophrenia into a full-blown psychosis. It can also exacerbate ongoing schizophrenia. This is really not surprising if we recall that the major tranquilizers so useful in treating schizophrenia block dopamine in the brain. Indeed, some believe that schizophrenia is a disorder of brain dopamine due to overproduction of dopamine or to an abnormal sensitivity of certain regions of the brain to dopamine.

An increase in the dosage in an attempt to gain better control of the symptoms may initiate a train of mental symptoms in patients who have been on long-term treatment. Vivid dreams and nightmares lead to insomnia. Sleep medications prove to be of little help and insomnia persists. Agitation and confusion occur during the day, followed by visual hallucinations, which are often dream-like in quality. This situation has been aptly termed the "dopa madness." Reversing it requires reducing the dosage of levodopa. In severe cases hospitalization for a drug holiday may be needed.

Depression or melancholia is not uncommon among parkinsonian patients. Some physicians have reported that levodopa may exacerbate or provoke depression. Others have thought it might help alleviate depression; most feel it has no effect. In our experience either effect may occur. Depression may be masked by the symptoms of parkinsonism, so that when the latter are relieved by levodopa treatment, the depression then becomes apparent. Therefore one should be alert to the possibility of depression. Effective treatment for depression is available and may be used in combination with levodopa therapy. Levodopa need not normally be discontinued. Usually both conditions can be treated simultaneously. Drugs commonly used to treat depression such as imipramine (Tofranil) and amitriptyline (Elavil) may readily be used at the same time as levodopa and may even work better with levodopa than if used alone. Some of the newer antidepressants work by inhibiting uptake of the neurotransmitter serotonin, thereby making it more available for use by brain cells. Common drugs in this group that can be used effectively by patients with Parkinson's disease are fluoxetine (Prozac), paroxetine (Paxil) and sertraline (Zoloft).

There is, however, one group of drugs sometimes used to treat depression that should never under any circumstances be given to a patient taking levodopa. This is the group of *monoamine oxidase (MAO) inhibitor* drugs. By blocking the action of the enzyme monoamine oxidase, these drugs turn off the body's normal mechanism for preventing excessive accumulation of dopamine, adrenaline and noradrenaline. Levodopa can be metabolized to all three of these substances, and so they accumulate very rapidly in abnormal amounts in the body if levodopa and a MAO inhibitor drug are taken together. The results are similar to the effects of an overdose of adrenaline. The heart pounds rapidly, the blood pressure shoots up very high, and palpitations, shortness of breath, nausea, vomiting, severe headaches, agitation, convulsions, and coma may result. There is a serious possibility of provoking a heart attack or a cerebral hemorrhage. Similar reactions can occur when a MAO inhibitor is combined with a variety of other drugs, such as amphetamine, and even with certain foods, especially cheddar cheese and certain wines. In fact since this reaction was first noted in patients who ate cheese while being treated with a MAO inhibitor, it has been called the "cheese reaction." The MAO inhibitor drugs in current use include pargyline (Eutonyl), phenelzine (Nardil), and tranylcypromine (Parnate).

LOW BLOOD PRESSURE

Levodopa also accumulates in other parts of the nervous system. It is believed to enter sympathetic nerves, which control the heart and blood vessels throughout the body. In these nerves levodopa simply enters the normal metabolic pathway for the formation of adrenaline and noradrenaline. However, because it is present in unnatural amounts, it may interfere with the normal function of the sympathetic nervous system. The result may be episodes of rapid heart beat (rapid pulse), which may be felt as palpitations. Elevation or depression of blood pressure may also occur. Indeed dopamine is now employed as a drug in its own right to treat low blood pressure; it is injected by vein to raise blood pressure as an emergency measure in patients with very low blood pressure following serious injuries or major surgery, a condition known as "shock." However, in patients taking levodopa the blood pressure usually tends to decrease. In fact in some patients it may fall to such low levels that symptoms such as faintness, dizziness, and lightheadedness result. Levodopa by mouth very rarely causes brief periods of high blood pressure. Low blood pressure is by far the most common side effect involving the circulatory system. A striking feature is that the blood pressure may be normal if measured in the lying or sitting position, only to fall when the patient stands up. This occurs because the blood pools in the legs. Normally the sympathetic nervous system acts on the blood vessels to counter the effects of gravity and maintain a uniform flow of blood to the head. This is accomplished by constriction of blood vessels in the legs, which prevents accumulation of blood in the leg muscles. The sympathetic nervous system is somewhat impaired in some patients with Parkinson's disease. The effect of levodopa on these nerves may further impair their function so that they may not be able to prevent the pooling of blood in the legs when the patient stands up.

This side effect of levodopa may be countered by several measures. A simple, frequently effective one is to administer salt tablets. Several tablets a day (containing 0.25 to 0.5 gram of sodium chloride) suffice for most patients having this side effect. Another measure is to wear elastic stockings to prevent blood pooling in the veins. This is especially useful in patients with varicose veins, which may pool a considerable volume of blood. A variety of such stockings are available, some ready-made, others made to order. The latter are more expensive but are also more effective and durable. Patients should put the stockings on in the morning before getting out of bed. Still another mechanical trick is to raise the head of the bed about 3 or 4 inches with wood blocks. This alters kidney function at night to cause increased salt retention.

If these countermeasures are not sufficient, the patient's physician may wish to try the drug fluorohydrocortisone. As the name implies, this drug is related to cortisone, the hormone of the adrenal cortex. Fluorohydrocortisone is a synthetic hormone that controls the metabolism of sodium chloride. It causes the kidney to retain more sodium chloride—and release less of it into the urine—than it would otherwise do. It is a very potent drug and has been helpful in the rare patient with severe low blood pressure complicating parkinsonism.

Midodrine is sometimes useful in Parkinson's disease patients with low blood pressure. This drug acts by stimulating the alpha-adrenergic receptors in the blood vessels, causing contraction, and thereby increasing pressure. Midodrine is still an investigational agent in the United States but can already be prescribed by physicians in a number of other countries under the name Gutron and Hipertan.

EFFECTS ON BLADDER AND BOWEL

Because the action of the bladder is under the influence of the sympathetic nerves, some weakening of bladder function is very occasionally experienced by patients when they first start levodopa treatment. The effect is relatively mild, indeed much milder than the similar effect of the anticholinergic drugs. It is a relatively rare side effect of levodopa and seems to occur only in men. Rarely patients report that they have more constipation on levodopa treatment, but there is no evidence that this is in fact a direct effect of the drug.

DISCOLORATION OF URINE AND SWEAT

A major portion of the levodopa absorbed by the intestine is removed from the circulation by the kidneys. The kidneys rapidly convert it to dopamine and then to a series of inactive substances. Some of these are pigments called melanins. They range in color from orange to red to brown and finally to black. The pigments are more likely to be formed if the urine is alkaline. Drops of urine reacting with alkaline materials, such as dried bleach in underclothing or bedsheets, may produce reddish or brownish stains. Many patients have been frightened by such stains, mistaking them for blood. Occasionally patients note after passing urine that the water in the toilet bowl is tinged with red. This is especially likely to occur if the bowl was recently treated with some disinfectant solution. In case of doubt it is best of course to consult a physician. The urine can very quickly be examined to ascertain whether there has been bleeding into the urinary tract.

A very small amount of levodopa may also be secreted by the sweat glands. Rarely, some dark beads of sweat result and stain undergarments.

INTERACTIONS WITH OTHER DRUGS

Patients are often concerned that a drug prescribed by another doctor for some acute illness may interfere with their levodopa. For example, they may have been given an antibiotic to treat the flu or some other infection. Or perhaps a doctor has prescribed an antihistamine to control some hay fever symptoms, or the dentist may want to administer Novocain before drilling. Many other examples come to mind. In nearly all of these situations, there is no problem. Levodopa is a particularly forgiving drug and can be used with almost anything. Only a few interactions of any significance have been encountered.

The number one "no-no" is to combine a monoamine oxidase (MAO) inhibitor drug with levodopa. We have already explained the potentially dangerous interactions that can occur when levodopa and a MAO inhibitor are taken together. Under no circumstances should these agents be combined.

MAO inhibitor drugs had been tried in the treatment of parkinsonism before the introduction of levodopa, but were soon abandoned as ineffective. They were tried again in combination with levodopa in the early days of experimentation with levodopa. The idea was to enhance and prolong the effect of levodopa. Although these drugs did enhance the effect of a given dose of levodopa, they did not prolong the duration of the response and, unfortunately, produced episodes of high blood pressure and very rapid pulse rates.

Aside from this one serious interaction, there is little to fear. All that can happen is that the effect of levodopa may be diminished. The major tranquilizer drugs, which act by blocking the action of dopamine in the nervous system, simply diminish the actions of levodopa. Therefore they should not be taken by patients on levodopa therapy. The drug metoclopramide (Reglan) employed to treat stomach disorders also blocks the action of dopamine and should be used cautiously if at all. Patients should also be cautious about taking vitamin preparations containing large amounts of vitamin B_6 (pyridoxine) because this vitamin can antagonize the effects of levodopa. The mechanism of this somewhat surprising interaction is explained in Chapter 10. Two calcium channel blockers (cinarrazine and flunarrazine) widely prescribed in Europe but not available in the United States may also block the effect of dopamine. These two drugs should be avoided by patients with Parkinson's disease. Other calcium channel blockers used to treat heart conditions or high blood pressure may rarely worsen the symptoms of parkinsonism. Since this side effect is so infrequent, however, these drugs may be employed without undue worry in the vast majority of patients.

There is no problem in giving antibiotics, analgesics, antihistamines, vaccines, flu shots, or Novocain anesthesia to Parkinson's disease patients on levodopa treatment.

ENZYME INHIBITOR DRUGS

Carbidopa and Benserazide

The conversion of L-dopa to dopamine (see page 63) is controlled by a specific enzyme bearing the impressive scientific name L-aromatic amino acid decarboxylase. When discussing levodopa metabolism, we commonly refer to this enzyme by the short name *dopa decarboxylase*. Several drugs inhibit this enzyme and are therefore known to the pharmacologist as dopa decarboxylase inhibitors. A few of these inhibitors greatly increase the effect of a given dose of levodopa in Parkinson patients, and two of them are used in combination with levodopa: carbidopa and benserazide. The combination of carbidopa and levodopa in a single tablet is marketed under the trade name Sinemet. A similar combination containing levodopa and benserazide (marketed under the name Madopar) is not available in the United States. Each of these formulations is available in several strengths (see Appendix 1). In our experience these two preparations are very similar in their effect.

These drugs modify the body's metabolism of levodopa by inhibiting dopa decarboxylase and thus preventing the conversion of levodopa to dopamine. The key to their value in treating parkinsonism is that they are unable to enter the brain. The brain differs from all other organs in having the ability to regulate the admission of substances traveling through the body in the circulation. It has in effect a highly selective barrier. We call it the blood–brain barrier. It admits levodopa but not dopamine. Similarly it does not admit carbidopa or benserazide. As a result of this curious circumstance, carbidopa and benserazide inhibit the conversion of levodopa to dopamine throughout the body *except* in the brain. Consequently these agents greatly increase the proportion of levodopa taken by mouth that ultimately reaches the brain and is converted to dopamine. In effect they protect the levodopa until it has a chance to reach the brain. The protection is not complete, but it is quite significant. In practice approximately 80% less levodopa needs to be taken by mouth when the combination treatment is used than when levodopa is used alone. This means that a patient who needs 5 grams of levodopa for symptom control now needs only 1 gram. Instead of ten 0.5-gram tablets of levodopa a day, an individual needs only four tablets of Sinemet or Madopar containing 0.25 gram of levodopa each. Taking four small pills instead of ten large ones is a matter of some convenience. However, the major bonus of combining levodopa with a decarboxylase inhibitor is that it largely abolishes the action of levodopa on the vomiting center. The reason for this is that this area does not hide behind the blood–brain barrier. To do its work, the vomiting center must be able to sample the various substances traveling in the circulation. Thus carbidopa and benserazide gain access to the vomiting center and prevent the formation of dopamine there.

The practical consequences of this situation are considerable. First, a patient just starting levodopa therapy need not begin with very small doses and build up slowly over a period of months to the full dosage while waiting for the vomiting center to develop tolerance for levodopa. Instead the patient can reach full dosage within a matter of days. Second, the various precautions discussed above to minimize levodopa-induced nausea and vomiting can now usually be ignored. Thus dose schedules can be set up in accord with the patient's need, without regard to mealtimes. The patient who requires levodopa immediately upon arising in the morning need not wait until after breakfast but can take the combination tablet even before getting out of bed. The patient who needs levodopa every 2 or 3 hours to maintain a smooth response throughout the day no longer needs to wait until the next meal but can take the combination tablet on an empty stomach. For these reasons treatment with Sinemet or Madopar is much more convenient and agreeable to both patient and physician. Levodopa is now rarely used alone.

It must be admitted of course that all is not perfect even in the most perfect of all possible worlds. There are still patients, though very few, who feel some nausea despite taking levodopa in combination with carbidopa or benserazide. These few patients must heed the precautions (discussed above) that were learned in the early days of levodopa therapy. One reason that the decarboxylase inhibitor may fail to protect all patients from activation of the vomiting center is that the amount of carbidopa in the lowest-strength Sinemet tablet may not be sufficient to prevent the formation of some dopamine in the vomiting center. The 10/100 Sinemet tablet contains 10 milligrams (mg) of carbidopa and 100 mg (or 0.10 gram) of levodopa. The obvious solution to this is to take an additional amount of carbidopa separately. This is provided in the 25/100 Sinemet tablet containing 25 mg of carbidopa. Because this tablet is scored, it is possible to use a half tablet, that is, 12.5/50 mg, and still have enough carbidopa to prevent nausea. Since the introduction of the 25/100 tablet, nausea has been a rare occurrence. Those rare patients who still have nausea may be helped by using diphenidol (Vontrol) or trimethobenzamide (Tigan).

If despite all these measures, nausea persists, one may have recourse to the drug metoclopramide (Reglan). Unfortunately metoclopramide blocks the action of dopamine not only in the stomach but also in the brain, and thus blocks the desired effects of levodopa treatment. Nevertheless, it can be used in low doses for a few weeks to ease the patient through this difficult period. The drug domperidone (Motilium), a cousin of metoclopramide, is more effective for this purpose and is routinely used in Europe and Canada to counter levodopa-induced nausea and stomach upsets. Unlike metoclopramide, it does not gain entry to the brain and thus does not risk blocking the desired effects of levodopa therapy on parkinsonism. Domperidone is not available in the United States; it can be obtained from pharmacists in Europe, Canada, Mexico, and elsewhere. A 10-mg tablet taken with each dose of levodopa/carbidopa can effectively block the nausea. The daily medication schedule may need to be adjusted so that both drugs are taken together. Protection against the vomiting effect of levodopa is greater if the protecting drug is taken simultaneously with levodopa, before the nausea and vomiting begin. When the feeling of nausea has developed, it is too late to expect much benefit from the protecting drug.

Selegiline

We have already emphasized the dangers of taking a monoamine oxidase (MAO) inhibitor along with levodopa. The combination risks inducing attacks of high blood pressure (the "cheese reaction"). However, the drug selegiline (Eldepryl)— a MAO inhibitor—is one very important exception to that warning; this drug is also known generically as deprenyl. The reason selegiline is an exception is that there are two types of the enzyme MAO: type A, present in the adrenal glands, heart, liver, and other organs; and type B, present in the brain. Dopamine in the brain is metabolized mainly by MAO-B. Selegiline inhibits MAO-B, but not MAO-A, and thus can safely be taken with levodopa.

Taken in combination with levodopa/carbidopa (Sinemet) or levodopa/benserazide (Madopar), selegiline enhances the effects of levodopa, both the good and the side effects. The standard dosage is one 5-mg tablet twice daily, one after breakfast and one after lunch. Because of its resemblance to amphetamine and a slight amphetamine-like action that might cause insomnia, patients are usually advised not to take it later in the day. Patients under our care have taken it after dinner or even at bedtime, with no effect on their sleep. Some patients seem to respond as well to one tablet a day. Higher daily dosages are not recommended because, at dosages above 10 mg per day, the selectivity for MAO-B inhibition may be lost and MAO-A inhibition may begin to occur, bringing the risk of hypertensive reactions.

In practice, the effects of adding selegiline to a Sinemet or Madopar regimen seem about the same as the effects that could be expected from increasing the dosage of levodopa 20 to 25%. Dyskinesias may become more pronounced. It may then be necessary to reduce the dose of levodopa by about that proportion. Because selegiline inhibits the breakdown of dopamine by MAO-B, it prolongs somewhat the duration of the benefit yielded by each dose of levodopa. Thus it is useful in patients who experience a wearing-off of levodopa between doses or on–off fluctuations. A moderate reduction in the fluctuations may be expected. In our experience it also improves the general quality of the response to levodopa treatment.

Selegiline seems to have few side effects of its own. The side effects are those of levodopa. Nausea is perhaps the most common side effect we have seen when adding selegiline to patients' Sinemet regimen. Usually this occurs in patients who experienced nausea earlier with Sinemet alone and is easily controlled by reducing the dose to half a tablet a day for a few weeks and then gradually building up to the standard dosage of two tablets daily. Again, the use of antinausea drugs such as diphenidol (Vontrol) or trimethobenzamide (Tigan) has occasionally been necessary, but tolerance to selegiline has usually developed fairly rapidly, with nausea subsiding in a month or two.

In addition to enhancing the effects of levodopa, selegiline may slightly lessen the symptoms of Parkinson's disease when given alone. In patients with newly diagnosed mild parkinsonism whose symptoms are bothersome but too minimal to require active treatment, selegiline can delay the need for levodopa therapy for months to a year or more. Accordingly, it is often recommended as the initial treatment of newly diagnosed Parkinson's disease. Sinemet or Madopar is then added when needed in the usual manner. This delaying effect on the need for levodopa was thought several years ago to indicate that selegiline has a retarding effect on the progression of Parkinson's disease. But with further experience, most physicians have come to believe that selegiline itself helps the symptoms of early Parkinson's disease without slowing the disease process itself.

8

Imitators of Dopamine

No one who can remember what parkinsonism was like before levodopa can doubt that it was a very great improvement over the drug treatments previously available. Great as this improvement was, however, levodopa was clearly not the final answer. From the earliest days of levodopa treatment, physicians have yearned for a still more effective drug. They have thought that some of the limitations of levodopa treatment stem from the fact that it has no effect itself but must first be converted to dopamine. For a number of theoretical reasons it has seemed desirable to find a substance that would not need to be converted to the active agent but could act the same way as dopamine. Some of the side effects of levodopa then might not occur.

Many drugs directly imitating the action of dopamine have been tested in Parkinson's disease patients. Two of these, bromocriptine (Parlodel) and pergolide (Permax) are now regularly used in the treatment of parkinsonism. More are in various stages of development. These "imitators" of dopamine are properly termed *dopamine receptor agonists*. To understand the meaning of this term, it is necessary to think for a moment about how dopamine works in the nervous system.

We have described dopamine as a chemical messenger essential to the normal function of the brain. It is the means whereby the nerve cells of the substantia nigra communicate with the corpus striatum. These nerve cells form and store dopamine; they release it in the corpus striatum. The nerve cells of the striatum receive this messenger at special receptor sites on their surfaces, which recognize and respond to dopamine but not to other naturally occurring chemical messengers. For example, the dopamine receptors will pay little attention to epinephrine, norepinephrine, serotonin, or other chemical messengers that are also normally present in the corpus striatum. They are highly specific for dopamine, and thus we may think of them as dopamine receptors.

Although the dopamine receptors are very selective regarding which chemical messengers they will recognize, they can be fooled. Many substances are now known to act at the dopamine receptors in much the same way dopamine does. Drugs that can activate a receptor are known collectively as "agonists" of that receptor, in contrast to those drugs that can block the receptor and are thus termed "antagonists."

The first dopamine receptor agonist to be tested in Parkinson patients was apomorphine. This drug has long been useful in medical practice as an emetic. It activates the dopamine receptors in the vomiting center and is used to induce vomiting. The late Dr. George Cotzias hypothesized that it might also act on the dopamine receptors in the corpus striatum and thereby control the symptoms of parkinsonism. In fact earlier, in the 1950s, it was reported by Dr. Albert Schwab in Boston that an injection of apomorphine temporarily reduced the tremor of Parkinson's disease. Dr. Cotzias gave apomorphine by mouth to a small number of patients in much the same way he had prescribed levodopa. That is, he started treatment with small doses that he gradually increased to allow his patients time to develop tolerance to the emetic action of apomorphine. With care and persistence he was able to reach substantial doses, and these did in fact yield significant relief of the symptoms of parkinsonism. He estimated that apomorphine was 40 to 50% as effective as levodopa. However, the blood tests he carried out in his patients indicated that there was a toxic effect on the kidneys. Cotzias and his colleagues searched for other drugs that might have the same properties. They tested a synthetic agent similar to apomorphine, *N*-methyl aporphine. The results were similar.

Although this work failed to produce a new treatment, it did show that a dopamine receptor agonist could have a significant anti-Parkinson effect; it also gave impetus to the search for better and less toxic agonists. A totally different drug, piribedil (Trivastal) was also found, somewhat unexpectedly, to be a dopamine receptor agonist. It too was tested in Parkinson patients but was abandoned as relatively ineffective. Then a synthetic analogue of ergotamine, the alkaloid drug used in treating migraine, was found to be a powerful dopamine receptor agonist. This drug, bromocriptine (Parlodel) appeared to have some advantages over levodopa in animal experiments. For example, its action lasted for 5 to 6 hours, whereas levodopa acted for only 2 to 3 hours in the same animals. It was also much more potent. A very small dose seemed equal in effect to a very large dose of levodopa.

Bromocriptine was initially tried in Parkinson patients by Dr. Donald Calne and his colleagues in London, England, in 1973. Definite effects were found with modest doses. These results were soon confirmed by other investigators. After a decade of extensive experimental treatment at various doses, alone and in combination with other drugs, bromocriptine became established as a useful addition to levodopa.

It is about 50% as effective as levodopa in relieving the symptoms of parkinsonism. Although it can be used alone in some patients for a period of time, it is most useful when used in combination with levodopa. Unfortunately it cannot fully substitute for levodopa. Probably the most important quality of this drug is that its action lasts longer than that of levodopa. It is thus most helpful in patients with the on–off effect who enjoy only a short-duration response from each dose of levodopa, even when taking it every 2 to 3 hours. Bromocriptine can reduce the fluctuations, making the "on" phases last longer and the "off" phases shorter and milder. It is especially useful for patients suffering painful muscle or "dystonic" cramps in their off phases.

The side effects are similar to those of levodopa. Loss of appetite, nausea, vomiting, lowering of blood pressure, involuntary movements, agitation, vivid dreams, nightmares, confusion, and hallucinations have all been reported. Tolerance to the nausea and vomiting takes place rapidly. Usually only mild nausea is encountered, and it subsides within a matter of days. Loss of appetite also disappears quickly and may be replaced by an increase in appetite after a period of time. A few patients have complained of gaining weight, but this has been minimal. Rarely blood pressure falls sufficiently to cause lightheadedness, dizziness, and faintness. It is also rare, but bromocriptine seems to activate long-quiescent peptic ulcer disease.

The major and most troublesome side effects have been mental disturbances. In the mildest cases the patient displays an unusual suspiciousness of loved ones and friends. This may be followed by anxiety, insomnia, and vivid dreams. If the drug is continued, episodes of confusion and visual hallucinations may develop. In the severest cases the patient is irrational and agitated. The propensity of bromocriptine to induce these toxic mental effects is greater than that of levodopa or the anticholinergic drugs. Of course, as with similar side effects with other drugs, these undesired manifestations subside rapidly after the drug is stopped.

Despite its side effects and limitations, bromocriptine (Parlodel) is a useful addition to the list of drugs now available to treat parkinsonism. It serves mainly as a supplement to levodopa. Used cautiously in specific situations, it can be very helpful. It is available in a 2.5-mg tablet and 5-mg capsule. Although some benefit may be seen with doses of 2.5 to 5 mg three times daily, larger doses of 10 to 20 mg three times daily, or even more, may be needed to obtain a significant effect. Treatment is usually begun with one half a 2.5-mg tablet at bedtime for 2 weeks to assure tolerance to the possible side effects. The dose is then increased to one half tablet three times daily after meals, later to a full tablet three times daily, and then to the 5-mg capsule three times daily. In this manner the dose can slowly be increased as needed. We rarely exceed a daily total of 40 mg.

Small doses of bromocriptine added to levodopa have been found to improve the quality of the response to treatment in mild cases of parkinsonism not experiencing the on–off effect. Professor Rinne of Turku University in Finland treated a group of patients with both bromocriptine and levodopa from the outset of treatment. He found that patients on the combined treatment fared better than those on levodopa alone over the 5 years of the study. Many neurologists initiate treatment with bromocriptine early in the course of the disease when the first indications of cramps or fluctuations in the response to levodopa emerge.

Another dopamine receptor agonist, pergolide (Permax), was studied extensively in the early 1980s in many centers in the United States and finally approved for use in Parkinson's disease in 1989. It is more potent than bromocriptine and thus is used in smaller doses. The benefits and side effects of the two drugs are very similar. In animal experiments the effects of pergolide last much longer than the effects of bromocriptine. One might thus expect that pergolide would be more help-ful in patients with the on–off effect, but in clinical practice there is no clear dif-ference between the two. When patients stop taking pergolide, the effects take 3 to 4 days to subside. It may then be necessary to increase the dose of levodopa to compensate for the loss of the beneficial effect of pergolide. Pergolide is available in 0.05-, 0.25- and 1.0-mg scored tablets, providing flexibility in adjusting the dosage. It is generally used in doses ranging from 0.25 to 2.0 mg three times daily.

Largely due to the work of Dr. Gerald Stern of the Middlesex Hospital, Lon-don, England, apomorphine has recently enjoyed renewed attention. Dr. Stern and his colleagues have developed its use in selected patients experiencing severe on–off fluctuations on levodopa therapy. The patients are trained to inject them-selves with a solution of apomorphine when they are in an off state. A prompt re-sponse occurs, lasting about 45 minutes. The patients use syringes and needles similar to those used to administer insulin to diabetics. Dr. Stern places his pa-tients on domperidone (Motilium) treatment to protect them from the nausea and vomiting that apomorphine might otherwise provoke. Some patients appear to benefit from this treatment. In our experience, however, only a few patients have found it worth the trouble and expense. The short duration of the response and the need to have the syringe and needle ready at the right moment limit its value. Apo-morphine is not readily available in the United States.

Another short-acting dopamine agonist is lisuride (marketed in Europe under the name Dopergine). Lisuride has been used in a water solution in a pump de-livering a solution of lisuride under the skin. Dr. José Obesso of Pamplona, Spain, pioneered the use of the lisuride pump in the management of severe on–off fluctuations.

Several dopamine receptor agonists are currently in clinical trials. These in-clude cabergoline, pramipexole and ropinerol. It is possible that one or more of these may prove superior to the ones now in regular use, but at the time of writ-ing they remain experimental drugs.

Over 40 dopamine receptor agonists have been tested in clinical trials over the past twenty years. Most have been abandoned because of toxic side effects. They all appear to have about the same degree of efficacy and similar side effects. None has shown sufficient efficacy to be used as the initial or as the only drug in the treatment of parkinsonism. None quite equals the action of levodopa. The reason is still not clear. Experiments in animal models of parkinsonism suggest that some effect of levodopa other than the replenishment of brain dopamine stores may be important. We emphasized in Chapter 1 the depletion of dopamine in parkinson-ism. There is also, however, a depletion of norepinephrine stores. Levodopa treat-ment may also, at least partially, correct the norepinephrine deficiency. The do-pamine receptor agonists do not activate the brain norepinephrine receptors.

Another possible explanation for the limited effects of the dopamine receptor agonists studied to date may lie in the fact that there are at least two major types of dopamine receptors. These have been designated the D-1 and D-2 receptors on the basis of certain distinct chemical properties. More recently additional subtypes have been identified. Thus we now have D-3 and D-4 receptors! Dopamine activates all these receptors. Bromocriptine activates only the D-2 receptor; it is actually an antagonist of the D-1 receptor! Pergolide is a weak D-1 and strong D-2 receptor agonist. Several selective D-1 agonists are presently known, but they are not available for use in patients. Studies by various investigators of D-1 receptor agonists in animals indicated that normal bodily movement requires activation of both types of receptors. However, limited trials in patients have not shown benefit when these are used alone or in combination with levodopa. The question remains open whether action at the D-1 receptor will be helpful to Parkinson's disease patients.

9

Special Remedies for Special Symptoms

In the preceding chapters we described the major anti-Parkinson drugs: the anticholinergics, levodopa, and the dopamine-receptor agonists. These drugs act on the parkinsonian state as a whole and are not directed specifically against any one symptom. In general they relieve all or at least most symptoms related to the classic triad: tremor, rigidity, and bradykinesia. There remains a miscellaneous group of drugs whose acquaintance many patients are apt to make sooner or later. They are not specific for parkinsonian symptoms but rather are used to treat symptoms that are very common such as insomnia, anxiety, constipation, etc. Some discussion of these drugs seems appropriate because Parkinson's disease patients may react differently to these commonly used agents, and some of these drugs may interact adversely with the major anti-Parkinson drugs.

PROPRANOLOL

The drug propranolol (Inderal) is used mainly to treat irregularity of the pulse and, to a lesser extent, to control high blood pressure. It may be used for these purposes in Parkinson patients with heart disease, irregular heart rate, or high blood pressure. It may also be used to protect the heart from the possibility of levodopa causing palpitations or episodes of abnormal heart rhythm in patients who are subject to palpitations.

Propranolol, however, has also been used occasionally because it seems to have a favorable effect on tremor, at least in some patients. Because the drug has an important action on the heart, it must be used with care. It is not recommended for patients who have asthma or have had heart failure since it may exacerbate these conditions.

Very occasionally a patient who still has some disturbing tremor despite good control of other symptoms of Parkinson's disease may enjoy a good response to this drug. Unfortunately propranolol has no effect on other symptoms.

Propranolol is commonly used to treat the symptom of tremor in the condition known as *benign essential tremor* or *familial tremor* (see Chapter 3). This is sometimes confused with parkinsonism because the tremor often bears a superficial resemblance. However, none of the other manifestations of Parkinson's disease develop in persons with essential or familial tremor, even after 40 to 50 years. On closer examination, their tremor differs in a number of respects from that of Parkinson's disease. One of these differences is that the tremor is not present at rest; instead it is present during movement or on maintaining a posture for a moment. Thus it is an action and a postural tremor. Another difference is that in essential tremor, the head and the voice are commonly involved; this rarely if ever occurs in Parkinson's disease. Finally, essential tremor responds differently to various drugs. In particular it can be suppressed for a few hours by alcohol, whereas the tremor of Parkinson's disease is not reduced by alcohol. A highball or a glass of sherry dramatically diminishes the former for a few hours but not the latter. The various minor tranquilizers may also effectively reduce essential tremor, paralleling the action of alcohol. Levodopa has no effect on essential tremor, but can greatly reduce or abolish the tremor of Parkinson's disease.

Several new drugs, closely related to propranolol, are available. One of these, metoprolol (Lopressor), is used primarily in treating high blood pressure. It is not as effective as propranolol against tremor, but has much less risk of exacerbating asthma.

MINOR TRANQUILIZERS AND HYPNOTICS

Minor tranquilizers are sometimes prescribed for patients with tremor persisting despite treatment with the usual anti-Parkinson drugs. They may also be given to relieve the sense of inner restlessness and nervousness that may occur as a symptom of Parkinson's disease or as a side effect of anti-Parkinson drugs. These symptoms most frequently occur when the effect of levodopa wears off between doses. It is better to deal with them by adjusting the doses or the schedule, or switching to a slow-release formulation, than to use tranquilizers. However, in some instances the mild tranquilizers may be helpful. Those most commonly used are lorazepam (Ativan), diazepam (Valium), oxazepam (Serax), and alprazolam (Xanax). These drugs are called "minor" tranquilizers to distinguish them from the "major" tranquilizers such as chlorpromazine (Thorazine), trifluoperazine (Stelazine), and haloperidol (Haldol), which are used primarily in psychiatric practice to treat severe mental illness. The major tranquilizers block the action of dopamine in the brain and consequently can cause parkinsonism. They therefore should not normally be given to Parkinson patients. The minor tranquilizers are entirely different and do not cause parkinsonism. They may in fact be quite useful but should be used sparingly and only as needed.

The minor tranquilizers can cause drowsiness, incoordination, dizziness, and confusion, and occasionally seem to increase the bradykinesia, or slowness of movement, of Parkinson's disease. Moreover, some persons may become psychologically dependent on or habituated to these drugs. Patients who use these drugs heavily for a period of time and then suddenly stop taking them may suffer withdrawal symptoms, including nervousness, agitation, and even (rarely) convulsions. However, we have never encountered a Parkinson patient who became dependent on these drugs, perhaps because we are careful to prescribe them sparingly.

What can the Parkinson patient with insomnia take to induce sleep? Preferably, of course, nothing. If levodopa (whether used alone or in a combined formulation with carbidopa or benserazide) seems to be responsible for insomnia, the bedtime dose should be avoided; if the drug is necessary, it might be reduced 50%. Several old nonmedical tricks may be quite helpful in inducing sleep at night, including a warm drink (such as a glass of warm milk) or even a brandy at bedtime. If insomnia is still a problem, a mild sedative such as chloral hydrate may be used. This is a very old and mild short-acting sedative that leaves no hangover and is least apt of all the available hypnotics to cause confusion. It is made in the form of 250- and 500-mg capsules. Usually one 500-mg capsule on retiring is successful, but another capsule may be taken an hour later if necessary. Two capsules (1.0 gram) may be used on retiring if one is not effective. A mild tranquilizer such as lorazepam (Ativan), 1 mg at bedtime, may also be helpful.

Parkinson patients more commonly have no trouble falling asleep on initially retiring. Rather their problem is that they wake up after several hours and then cannot get to sleep again. If there are recurrent Parkinson symptoms at that time—stiffness, cramps, or just slowness—and the patient cannot find a comfortable position, then an additional dose of levodopa/carbidopa (Sinemet) or levodopa/benserazide (Madopar) may be helpful. Using a slow-release preparation such as Sinemet CR or Madopar HBS at bedtime will often provide an extra hour or two of sleep by delaying the wearing-off that causes the patient to wake up.

The drugs flurazepam (Dalmane) and temazepam (Restoril) are commonly prescribed hypnotics. They are closely related to diazepam (Valium) and may also increase the bradykinesia of parkinsonism. Thus we generally avoid these drugs in treating our patients.

TREATMENT OF HALLUCINATIONS AND PARANOIA

Since the advent of levodopa therapy, most patients with Parkinson's disease are living longer. Consequently more patients are encountering some of the complications of advancing disease. Dr. Christopher Goetz and his colleagues at Rush–Presbyterian–St. Luke's Medical Center in Chicago have emphasized that the presence of hallucinations or paranoia is the single most important factor determining whether a Parkinson patient will need long-term nursing home care. It is therefore important to keep these symptoms controlled. As discussed in Chapter 8, levodopa can sometimes provoke hallucinations or paranoia. The other drugs used to treat parkinsonism in conjunction with levodopa, however, are even more prone to exacerbate these mental aberrations.

Many steps taken to reduce hallucinations and paranoia inevitably worsen the motor symptoms of Parkinson's disease. Initially, decreasing the secondary drugs may control hallucinations and paranoia. Selegiline (Eldepryl), anticholinergic drugs, and dopamine-receptor agonists are discontinued one at a time. Most patients and spouses willingly trade lessened psychotic behavior for more tremor or slowness. Sometimes small doses of the major tranquilizers discussed in the previous section can reduce hallucinations or paranoia; these drugs are rarely helpful for very long and can exacerbate the parkinsonism. Over the past several years, Dr. Joseph Friedman at Brown University and others have advocated the use of clozapine (Clozaril) to treat psychosis associated with parkinsonism. This drug blocks the effect of dopamine mostly in the limbic system and cortex (the part of the brain responsible for hallucinations) and has less effect on dopamine in the corpus striatum. It therefore does not worsen the symptoms of Parkinson's disease. Unfortunately clozapine can be dangerous since it may depress neutrophils (white blood cells) to critical levels. All patients on clozapine are required to undergo weekly blood tests, and the drug must be stopped if the number of neutrophils drops below the danger point.

OVER-THE-COUNTER SEDATIVES

Parkinson patients should avoid over-the-counter sedatives such as Compoz, Sominex, Sleep-eze, Nytol, and others. These preparations all contain scopolamine (hyoscine) as an active ingredient, in quantities comparable to those formerly employed in treating parkinsonism (see the discussion of solanaceous alkaloids in Chapter 6). They also contain an over-the-counter antihistamine, methapyrilene hydrochloride, which like other antihistamines also has some anticholinergic activity. The addition of these agents to a Parkinson patient's existing drug regimen, which may already include some anticholinergic agents, may carry the patient over the threshold of anticholinergic toxicity. Consequently Parkinson patients are less able to tolerate the side effects commonly produced by these medications. On the other hand, the anticholinergic properties of these formulations may have some beneficial effect on the symptoms of parkinsonism. Patients should consult their doctors before trying them, however, to minimize the chance of an unpleasant interaction with their own anti-Parkinson drug treatment.

DIURETICS

Swelling of the feet due to the accumulation of water in the tissues (edema) of the legs and feet is a common manifestation of parkinsonism. It is often more marked in one leg, nearly always the leg on the side where the first symptoms occurred. The causes of this swelling are not fully understood. One reason may be that there is less muscular activity in that limb due to the bradykinesia of parkinsonism. In any event the swelling can be relieved by diuretic agents (that is, drugs that increase the volume of urine passed in a day). Milder diuretics such as hydrochlorothiazide (Hydrodiuril) may effectively relieve this swelling. Usually only one dose once or twice a week is necessary. The drug should be taken only with a doctor's prescription.

If the swelling was induced by the drug amantadine (Symmetrel), it should subside when that drug is stopped, although it may require several weeks to disappear. If varicose veins are present, elastic hose may be helpful. Further treatment may be advised by the doctor.

LAXATIVES

Chronic constipation is a familiar symptom of Parkinson's disease. It results from a general slowing of the muscular action of the bowel or of muscular action in other organs. As mentioned earlier, constipation is also often exacerbated by the drugs used in treating parkinsonism. The tendency of Parkinson patients to drink little water is a further complicating factor. Consequently many patients need to take laxatives.

We urge patients to try natural means of maintaining normal bowel habits. This means making an effort to drink more water, to eat adequate roughage and high-fiber foods, and to ingest prunes, prune juice, or figs regularly. A favorite regimen is stewed prunes, bran cereal, and apple sauce for breakfast. Failing all this, one must resort to laxatives. Several classes of laxatives need be considered.

First, there are bulk laxatives that work by retaining water in the stools. Patients who pass small, hard stools—really dehydrated stools—may benefit from this measure alone. A common laxative in this class is Metamucil, available over the counter. A tablespoonful stirred in one glass of water a day may suffice.

Another useful preparation is the fecal softener dioctyl sodium sulfosuccinate (also known as docusate sodium). A great many proprietary over-the-counter preparations containing this ingredient are available. One capsule one, two, or three times daily may be used. Generally these are used on a regular daily maintenance basis by Parkinson patients.

If these measures are inadequate, an "irritant" laxative that stimulates the bowel directly may be required. Milder ones such as bisacodyl (Dulcolax) are preferable. Some preparations combine such a stimulant with the fecal softeners mentioned above. The pharmacist can give advice about a suitable one, or the patient can check the label on the packages on the supermarket shelf, looking for the two ingredients dioctyl sodium sulfosuccinate (docusate sodium) and bisacodyl. We have also found lactulose helpful in some cases of severe constipation. We have found that cisapride (Propulsid) may also alleviate constipation in many patients with Parkinson's disease without causing undue side effects such as diarrhea. This drug increases the movement of stool through the colon by stimulating the nerves to the intestine. It must be prescribed by a physician

Finally many patients have a laxative habit acquired long before Parkinson's disease developed. They may prefer to continue using their old favorites. As a last resort enemas may be required to maintain adequate evacuation. ·

ARTIFICIAL TEARS

The reduced frequency of spontaneous eye blink that is common in parkinsonism may result in some redness and dryness of the eyes and eyelids. The lids may become encrusted. Patients feel some irritation, a dry, burning feeling in the eyes. Usually the major anti-Parkinson drugs restore eye blink to more normal frequency; with improvement in the normal "windshield wiper" function of the eyelids, these symptoms are relieved. However, if there is still some eye discomfort, irrigating the eyes with artificial tear solutions may be helpful. Various preparations of artificial tears can be purchased at local drug stores over the counter. They reproduce the salt concentration of natural tears. If symptoms are not relieved by this simple measure, medical advice should be sought.

TREATMENT FOR SEBORRHEA

The increased activity of the sebaceous glands of the skin in patients with Parkinson's disease commonly results in a somewhat greasy appearance of the face and forehead (seborrhea); occasionally, some have irritation and inflammation of the skin (seborrheic dermatitis). The seborrhea and the secondary dermatitis are reduced by treatment, especially by levodopa, and are rarely serious problems. To prevent the irritation, the oily secretion should be removed daily by washing the affected areas with a bland or neutral soap, with gentle scrubbing using an abrasive sponge or a face cloth. A commonly used soap formulation is the acne aid bar available at most drug stores. Dermatitis responds to a variety of lotions containing small amounts of hydrocortisone or related agents, but these require a doctor's prescription. Lotions, however, will seal in the irritating oily secretions of the skin, and so they should be applied after washing or scrubbing the affected areas.

A variety of hair lotions are available over the counter that may satisfactorily control excessive dandruff. One of the more effective contains selenium and is marketed under the name Selsun. A more concentrated solution of selenium is also available with a doctor's prescription. Many authorities advise that selenium preparations be used sparingly because they may cause hair loss if used excessively. It would be preferable to reserve them as a last resort and then use them only occasionally.

DRUGS FOR LEG CRAMPS

Foot and leg cramps are a bona fide Parkinson's disease symptom, although rarely the initial symptom of the disease. They are most often due to wearing off of the levodopa benefit. Typically they occur early in the morning when patients first get out of bed, but may also occur, or recur, during the day as the "dopa effect" wears off between doses. This "end-of-dose" dystonia is associated with spasm of the muscles of the calf and sole of the foot, in-turning of the foot, and clawing of the toes. Measures to counteract motor fluctuations generally alleviate or prevent these cramps. These include giving additional doses of levodopa/carbidopa (Sinemet) or levodopa/benserazide (Madopar), changing to a slow-release formulation (Sinemet CR; Madopar HBS), or adding a secondary anti-Parkinson drug. The dopamine-receptor agonists, bromocriptine (Parlodel) and pergolide (Permax), are the most effective in combating these cramps. One may also try baclofen (Lioresal) at the recommended dosage of 10 mg three times daily. Double this amount, however, may be needed to yield substantial relief. Some individuals have difficulty tolerating these doses of baclofen owing to nausea, dizziness, and drowsiness. Vitamin E (alpha-tocopherol) has been recommended by some physicians to prevent nocturnal cramps, but it has not been effective in our patients.

10

Surgical Treatment of Parkinsonism

The surgical treatment of Parkinson's disease received a lot of attention in the 1950s and the 1960s. A variety of surgical procedures was rapidly developed during those years at medical centers throughout the world. With the advent of levodopa in 1968–1970, the surgical treatment of parkinsonism was suddenly largely abandoned. The benefits of levodopa treatment were so remarkable in comparison with the effects achieved with our best previous medical treatment that surgery was reserved only for those patients who tolerated levodopa poorly or had persistent tremor despite optimal drug treatment. As a result the number of operations performed fell sharply, and many surgeons stopped performing the procedure altogether.

A few neurologists and neurosurgeons, however, continued to offer the procedure and gradually improved the techniques. New imaging methods such as computerized x-ray tomography (called the CAT or CT scan) and magnetic resonance imaging (MRI), developed in the 1980s, and computers capable of rapidly carrying out the necessary geometrical calculations have made a surgical technique called stereotactic surgery simpler and more precise. Recently better understanding of the basal ganglia and the effects of precisely placed lesions in the brain have sparked a renewed interest in brain surgery for parkinsonism. Although it is in no sense a cure and is useful in only a relatively small number of patients, modern brain surgery has a definite, if limited, place in the treatment of parkinsonism.

The first surgical efforts to alleviate parkinsonism were made during the 1930s. Various destructive operations were carried out in which some region of the cerebral cortex was removed or fibers deep in the brain were cut. The idea, stated somewhat crudely, was simply to damage the motor pathways enough to diminish tremor and rigidity without causing appreciable weakness. The results were mediocre and unpredictable, and the operations were relatively hazardous. Better procedures gradually evolved, largely from thoughtful trial and error and astute observation of accidental results. Dr. Russell Myers, a neurosurgeon then working at the Long Island College Hospital in New York, made an interesting discovery in 1939 while operating on a Parkinson patient with a brain tumor. When he cut through a part of the corpus striatum, tremor and rigidity on the opposite side of the body suddenly diminished. Taking advantage of this chance observation, he repeated the procedure in several more Parkinson patients. After trying a number of modifications based on the knowledge of brain anatomy available at the time, he found that the best effect could be achieved by severing a very small bundle of nerve fibers, deep in the brain, called the "ansa lenticularis." This bundle could be severed without producing any apparent ill effect, and the result was an appreciable reduction of tremor and rigidity in some patients. It was, however, very difficult to reach a small fiber bundle deep in the brain with a scalpel, without inflicting damage to other brain structures. Complications were serious and frequent, and few operations were actually done.

Many surgeons around the world tried to solve the problem of cutting that small fiber bundle safely and effectively. The most successful procedure turned out to be a technique known as *stereotactic surgery*. The technique had long been employed in experimental brain surgery in animals. Drs. Henry T. Wycis and Ernest Spiegel, working at Temple University Hospital in Philadelphia, and Dr. Hiro Narabayashi, working independently in Tokyo, adapted this technique to human patients in 1948. They lowered a long needle-like probe into the brain through a small burr hole in the overlying skull. The direction and depth of the needle was carefully calculated from landmarks located on x-ray films of the patient's head. Placing the probe in the desired place was a simple problem in spatial or three-dimensional geometry, and it could be done with considerable precision. When the probe was positioned satisfactorily, a solution of alcohol could be injected or an electrical current run from its tip, thereby destroying a small amount of brain tissue and severing the nerve fiber bundle. Drs. Wycis and Spiegel called their operation "ansotomy."

That small nerve fiber bundle identified as the target by Dr. Myers back in 1939 connects a structure called the *globus pallidum* (from the Latin, meaning pale body) to another called the *thalamus*. Some surgeons chose the pallidum as their target. The operation was called "pallidotomy." Others chose the termination of those fibers in the thalamus, calling their operation "thalamotomy." Similar results were obtained by all three procedures. With the technology available in the 1960s, it was easier to locate the thalamus, and the results appeared to be better and the side effects less frequent and less severe than with pallidotomy. Thus thalamotomy became the standard stereotactic operation for parkinsonism.

Various techniques of stereotactic surgery were developed. One that received much publicity was the cryosurgery technique developed by the late Dr. Irving Cooper at St. Barnabas Hospital in New York in the 1960s. Dr. Cooper used a needle with a system of tiny tubes through which a refrigerant solution of liquid nitrogen could be pumped. The effect was to freeze a small area of brain. Most stereotactic surgeons, however, used a radiofrequency current delivered from the tip of the stereotactic probe. The probe could also be used to record the electrical activity of the brain tissue through which it passed on the way to the target. This electrophysiological recording became a valuable aid to accurate placement of the needle. With such refinements in technique, the stereotactic surgeons were able to limit the damage to a very small volume of brain tissue, of the order of several cubic millimeters. In experienced hands such as those of Dr. Narabayashi, extremely precise operations were possible, tailored precisely to the needs of the individual patient.

These techniques were used to operate on many thousands of patients at special centers throughout the world. Although these operations effectively reduced tremor and rigidity on one side of the body in most cases, they nevertheless stirred considerable controversy. No one could satisfactorily explain why the operations worked. Many thoughtful physicians were disturbed by the idea of treating a disease whose symptoms reflected some poorly understood brain dysfunction by injuring the brain and causing further change in function, which was also poorly understood. Brain surgery could not cure or even alter the future progress of Parkinson's disease, and it relieved only some symptoms, mainly tremor and rigidity. Moreover, the operation had to be done twice, once for each side, if the symptoms on both sides of the body were to be relieved; and complications were much more frequent when both sides were operated on.

The major risk of stereotactic brain surgery was the possibility that the needle, pushed blindly through the brain toward the desired target, might injure a blood vessel and cause bleeding or clotting. The result would in effect be a stroke. There was also some difficulty because the standard measurement did not apply to all individuals, and as a result the needle might be placed a few millimeters off the target. Weakness of the arm or leg occasionally resulted, and in some the operation failed to give appreciable or lasting relief of tremor.

With experienced neurosurgeons the results were generally good and the risks relatively small. The chance of dying as a result of the operation was less than 1%. There was a 2 to 3% chance of some permanent weakness of the hand or leg on one side. Tremor and rigidity were markedly alleviated in 70 to 80% of cases. The results were less favorable when the second side was operated on. Especially troublesome was the development of slurring of speech and difficulty swallowing after the second operation. This occurred in as many as 15 to 20% of patients who were operated on twice.

To minimize risks, the surgeons were cautious in choosing patients on whom to operate. Not surprisingly the best results were obtained in young patients whose symptoms were mainly on one side and who were in good general health. Complications were more frequent in the elderly and especially in patients who had high blood pressure, diabetes, arteriosclerosis, heart disease, or other disorders affecting general health. It was also found that patients who had severe bradykinesia were not as likely to benefit from the operation as those who had only tremor and rigidity. Impairment of equilibrium during walking was not helped and sometimes was made worse. Speech dysfunction was not improved by surgery. Patients who were severely affected with Parkinson's disease were not likely to experience improvement.

As the neurosurgeons who specialized in this type of surgery gained experience, they narrowed their criteria for selecting patients for surgery. The criteria eventually became rather strict so that even the most aggressive and enthusiastic surgeons found only approximately 10% of Parkinson patients suitable for surgery. In the remaining 90% the risks of surgery were considered too great and the likelihood of real benefit too small. Thus despite all the publicity it received, stereotactic surgery was rather disappointing for many patients and their doctors.

There is no denying that stereotactic surgery did help many patients and that the results were occasionally dramatic. The operations were performed under local anesthesia with the patient awake throughout the procedure. Many patients described with wonderment and awe how they felt when the tremor suddenly stopped during the surgery. An excellent subjective account was given by the late Margaret Bourke White, a famous photographer. She wrote magazine articles and later a book about her experience of Parkinson's disease and her operation.

The publicity the operations received as a result of such individual accounts was a frequent cause of disappointment to the many patients who were not considered suitable for surgery. They had been led to hope for a miraculous cure by uncritical reports that appeared frequently in the popular press and in television documentaries. They sometimes had difficulty understanding why they too could not be helped. Many patients who were operated on and enjoyed good relief of tremor and rigidity were also disappointed when similar symptoms appeared in the opposite limbs several years later. They had hoped that the operation would cure the disease or at least prevent its further progression. But in fact stereotactic surgery was nothing more than a symptomatic remedy for tremor and rigidity. It was not specific for Parkinson's disease but could alleviate these symptoms in many other conditions. Indeed it is especially effective in relieving essential tremor.

In the past decade the earlier pallidotomy procedure has received renewed attention due to the work of Dr. L. Laitinen in Sweden and Dr. Mahlon DeLong at Emory University in Atlanta, Georgia. Dr. Laitinen felt that the operation relieved not only tremor and rigidity but also to some extent bradykinesia. Dr. DeLong's studies of the physiology of the basal ganglia in monkeys have given us new insight into the workings of this mysterious part of the brain and its dysfunction in Parkinson's disease. His work led him to the conclusion that pallidotomy was more effective then thalamotomy. He developed a new approach, based on careful recording of electrical activity in the pallidum, that defines the area of greatest abnormality within the pallidum; the object of surgery then is to destroy that small region. His data show that without the electrical recording, one can miss the area of abnormal activity and thus fail to do much good for the patient. This work has stimulated renewed interest in stereotactic brain surgery in the treatment of parkinsonism. As a result pallidotomy is now being offered at a number of centers. Although the number of patients undergoing this new technique is not yet very large, the results do appear to be useful in well selected cases. Our observation is that pallidotomy can help some patients. The results are similar to those provided by thalamotomy, but it is not clear that the results are better than those obtained with thalamotomy.

It is important to realize that pallidotomy is not a treatment for parkinsonism generally to be used in all patients. It is most useful in dealing with certain symptoms that do not respond to or are made worse by drug treatment (see the case of Mrs. S. below). In rare cases, painful muscle spasms may develop in a leg or arm and worsen with continued drug treatment. These spasms prevent the patient from getting a good effect from drug treatment. Pallidotomy can relieve these spasms and allow the patient to obtain better results from anti-Parkinson medications. But pallidotomy will not benefit patients unable to stand or walk due to lack of equilibrium or patients with extreme slowness of movement.

Dr. Jean Siegfreid of Zurich, Switzerland, Dr. Alim Benabid of Grenoble, France, and others have studied the effects of direct electrical stimulation of the thalamus in the treatment of essential tremor and parkinsonism. They implant a fine wire electrode into the desired region of the thalamus. The wire is left in place and connected to a battery-driven stimulator. The idea is that high frequency stimulation of the thalamus may "jam" the nerve circuits involved and thus mimic the effects of thalamotomy. Early results appear interesting, but this procedure should still be considered experimental.

Many patients who may be expected to benefit from an operation choose not to undergo surgery. It is a personal choice that should be made rationally with full understanding of the possible benefits and risks. An example is a long-time patient, Mrs. S., a pleasant 55-year-old woman who had a mild resting tremor in her left hand and foot. It did not interfere with her life or her work as a cashier. The tremor disappeared with levodopa treatment only to be replaced by constant involuntary writhing movements of the left hand and foot, which Mrs. S. found just as disagreeable as the tremor. Other medications gave only slight relief. After trying various doses and schedules, she finally decided to give up on levodopa. The involuntary movements stopped, but the tremor recurred exactly as before. Twenty years after her tremor first appeared, she still had no symptom other than tremor of her left hand and foot. It had become slightly more prominent over the years and at times affected her chin, but there was no tremor on the right side or other symptoms of Parkinson's disease. Mrs. S. retired at age 70 and subsequently lived a happy and very active life doing the many things she had dreamed of doing during the years she was working. She remained unwilling to have brain surgery even though chances are very good that her tremor could have been abolished.

Mrs. S. illustrates an important limitation of stereotactic surgery in the treatment of parkinsonism. The one symptom that this surgery can most effectively relieve, regardless of its cause, is tremor, but patients who have only tremor and no other symptoms are rarely interested in having brain surgery. It is later in the course of Parkinson's disease, when slowness of movement, poor equilibrium, difficulty walking, and other, more disturbing symptoms appear that most patients are willing to undergo surgery. Unfortunately these more serious symptoms are not appreciably helped by stereotactic surgery—and may even be made worse. Thus when the patients really need help, surgery is not effective. Although thalamotomy or pallidotomy would almost certainly have benefited Mrs. S., one cannot argue with her decision. It was hers to make, and she remained confident that she made the right choice.

BRAIN TRANSPLANTS

The surgical treatment of Parkinson's disease took a new twist in the 1980s with attempts to transplant dopamine-producing nerve cells into the corpus striatum. The idea was to replace the lost dopamine-producing nerve cells of the substantia nigra with new ones placed directly in the striatum where the substantia nigra nerve cells normally deliver their dopamine. One source of such cells is the adrenal gland. Although the cells of the adrenal gland chiefly produce adrenaline (epinephrine), they also produce some dopamine. A better source of dopamine-producing nerve cells is the region of the midbrain where the substantia nigra is located. Using a microscope, researchers were able to dissect out this region from fetal or newborn animals and transplant it into the striatum of an adult animal. The nerve cells in these transplants survived, grew, and proved capable of at least partially correcting experimentally induced parkinsonism in rats, marmosets, and monkeys.

Building on this experience with transplants in rats, a Swedish group attempted adrenal-to-brain transplants in 4 Parkinson's disease patients in 1981–1984. The results were disappointing, and they concluded that this approach held little promise. However, a neurosurgeon in Mexico, Dr. Ignaccio Madrazzo, reported dramatic benefits with adrenal transplants in human patients. The first two patients were young, 33 and 35 years of age, and their parkinsonism atypical so that it was not clear what disease they had. One patient did so well that he no longer needed levodopa! Dr. Madrazzo's reports stirred great interest, and within a year a number of American surgeons also attempted adrenal transplants in Parkinson patients. They thought that perhaps some differences in technique might have accounted for the better results reported by the Mexican surgeon. Within a short time several hundred patients had this surgery. However, the procedure required two major operations performed one immediately after the other: the first to remove an adrenal gland and then a second operation on the head to implant a portion of the gland into the striatum. This was a considerable stress on older patients weakened by Parkinson's disease. Not surprisingly there were a substantial number of serious complications and some deaths. The results proved disappointing. No one could reproduce the dramatic initial results claimed by Madrazzo. The reason became apparent when several patients were subsequently studied postmortem. It was found that the transplanted adrenal nerve cells had not survived. The pathologists found a mass of dead and dying adrenal cells surrounded by inflammatory cells at the transplant site.

Both the initial claims of success and the subsequent disappointment received wide coverage in the public media. The American Academy of Neurology and other organizations called for a halt to the transplant operations until the results could be fully evaluated. A careful follow-up evaluation of a large number of cases in 1989 by a group of neurologists led by Dr. Christopher Goetz of the Rush–Presbyterian–St. Luke's Medical Center in Chicago, Dr. Warren Olanow of the University of South Florida, and Dr. William Koller of the University of Kansas found that benefits had been minimal and were not sustained. Adrenal transplants were abandoned.

FETAL-TISSUE TRANSPLANTS

Meanwhile a Swedish group led by Dr. Olle Lindval at the University of Lund began a long-term study of the effects of human fetal-cell transplants in human patients in a careful and methodical manner. They operated on their first patient in 1987 and the second in 1988. They have since proceeded very slowly, carefully evaluating the results and improving their techniques at each step. They early learned that the best results occurred when the transplant was placed in the region of the striatum called the putamen. This is the region where the loss of dopamine is the greatest in Parkinson's disease. All patients were also treated with drugs to suppress the immune system.

At this time, after 7 years, they have operated on only 16 patients including two who had parkinsonism induced by N-methylphenyl tetrahydropyridine (MPTP), a contaminant in illicit "street" drugs. Dr. Lindval reported the results at the third international meeting of the Movement Disorders Society in Orlando, Florida, in December 1994. This was the most extensive assessment then available of the possibilities of this type of transplant surgery. Improvements first appeared about 5 to 6 months after the operation and continued for up to 2 to 5 years. Improvement in on–off fluctuations with increased "on" time and less severe "off" periods was observed in 5 of the first 10 patients. Gait impairments were improved in 2 patients. One patient showed no response to the surgery, and Dr. Lindval believes the diagnosis of Parkinson's disease was probably incorrect. A reduction in levodopa dosage was possible in some cases. However, new symptoms also appeared, reflecting progression of the disease. Most patients had the transplant surgery on only one side of the brain, so the improvements were seen on the opposite side of the body; Parkinson symptoms continued to progress on the same side of the body as the surgery was performed. Poor balance developed in one patient, and as we have noted, this symptom is not always responsive to levodopa treatment and may not be due to dopamine deficiency.

In a second series of patients, Dr. Lindval and his team are transplanting more fetal tissue into both sides of the brain and in up to 7 different sites in different parts of the striatum. These more recent operations require a larger number of donor fetuses (from 4 to 7) to obtain sufficient tissue.

In an international collaboration these Swedish patients were studied each year at the Hammersmith Hospital, London, England, to check on the progress of the graft. The studies involved an imaging method known as positron emission tomography (PET) (more fully described on pages 142–143). The PET scans have shown that the transplanted cells survive and are able to take up levodopa and convert it to dopamine. Repeat PET scans showed that the transplants grew slowly and then remained about the same size 3 to 4 years after the transplantation. However, the scans also showed that the patients' own dopamine systems deteriorated during this period. The dopamine cells in the graft are apparently doing well, but the patients' own dopamine brain cells continue to deteriorate as expected. This indicates that whatever causes dopamine nerve cells to deteriorate does not affect the grafted cells.

A number of other surgical teams have attempted fetal brain transplants. At this time about 200 operations have been done worldwide, but few have been well monitored and the results have not yet been fully reported in scientific or medical journals. In 1986 a neurological group at Yale University, headed by Dr. Redmond and Dr. Kenneth Marek, initiated a fetal-cell transplant program that included plans to operate on 20 patients. So far only 9 patients have had surgery. Another group, led by Dr. Curt Freed, at the University of Colorado has operated on a number of patients and is now collaborating in a study sponsored by the National Institutes of Health (NIH) to assess the benefits of the transplant procedure in 40 patients. The patients will have the surgery at the University of Colorado but will be studied in New York at Columbia University. One half the study patients will have a sham procedure. That is, an operation will be done but no graft will be implanted. Neither the evaluating doctors nor the patients will know which patients received the graft. Both will thus be "blind" to the treatment given. This "double-blind" procedure will assure an objective assessment of the benefits, if any, of the graft procedure.

It should be clear that fetal-cell transplants remain an experimental treatment still in an early stage of development. A full assessment of its effects remains some years away. However, we can conclude from the available reports that dopamine cell transplants appear to be effective only in patients who are responsive to levodopa therapy but have severe on–off fluctuations. Patients not responsive to levodopa are not likely to be helped. Benefits begin to appear 5 to 6 months after the operation, increase for a period of time, and then appear to be maintained for periods of up to several years. Relief of symptoms has been only partial. How long the benefits will be maintained is not yet known. However, because the disease continues to progress, the later development of symptoms not related to dopamine deficiency, and thus not responsive to levodopa therapy, may eventually offset any benefits gained by surgery. The transplants are in no sense a cure.

Many technical aspects of the transplant procedure require further research. One of these is the question whether the transplant patient's immune system needs to be suppressed to prevent rejection of the transplanted tissue. To reduce that possibility, Dr. Lindval's group has treated patients with immunosuppressant drugs like those used in heart and kidney transplant patients. No one yet knows whether or for how long immunosuppression is necessary. Nor are the risks of long-term immunosuppression fully known in the Parkinson patient. Some groups are not using immunosuppressants or are using them in some patients but not in others to test whether they make a difference. Further investigation is also needed to determine the ideal size, number, and locations of the transplants. Perhaps these need to be adjusted to each patient's particular symptoms. Dr. Lindval suggests that transplant of noradrenaline-producing cells may also be important. This has not yet been tried.

Difficult ethical and troubling moral questions surround the use of living human tissue obtained from aborted fetuses. Guidelines have been formulated by various scientific and professional bodies for the procurement, handling, and use of human fetal tissue. They draw from the guidelines developed over many years for human organ transplants. However, the use of fetal tissue is not strictly comparable to collecting organs from brain-dead patients or cadavers. Since fetal tissue can only be acquired from aborted fetuses, many find the approach morally unacceptable. The ethical and moral objections to the use of fetal cells could be circumvented by using artificial or genetically engineered cells maintained in tissue cultures. Many "lines" of such cells exist and some have already been shown to alleviate parkinsonism in animals with MPTP-induced parkinsonism. Such cells have not yet been transplanted into human patients.

Dr. Lindval emphasizes that at present fetal-cell transplantation is an experimental procedure. Asked when he expects fetal-cell grafts may become a treatment for Parkinson's disease, he cautiously places the time 10 to 15 years into the future. We believe that advances in other areas, especially the genetic aspects of Parkinson's disease, will lead to entirely new and far more effective treatments before then.

11

Dietary Considerations

Malnutrition can cause disturbances—even very serious disturbances—of the nervous system, including various paralyses, loss of feeling, incoordination, convulsions, and mental deterioration; but malnutrition has never caused parkinsonism. There is no known nutritional deficiency responsible for or characteristic of parkinsonism.

Nor, aside from levodopa, is there any known food or special nutrient, vitamin, or mineral that has a therapeutic effect. Consequently there is no dietary treatment. Contrary to what one may read in magazine articles or popular books on nutrition, there is no diet or food that is known to have a beneficial effect on the symptoms of Parkinson's disease or other forms of parkinsonism.

The best dietary advice for patients with parkinsonism is to eat as normally as possible. The patient should attend to his or her general health and should eat a well-balanced diet with fruits, vegetables, adequate protein, roughage, cereal, etc.

Since a tendency to constipation is common in Parkinson patients, special attention to roughage and natural laxatives is warranted. Many patients find it beneficial to eat prunes or figs regularly. Roughage and high-fiber foods such as carrots, cauliflower, broccoli, bran cereals, etc. are helpful in increasing the bulk of the stool. Patients who tend to have small, hard, "rock-like" stools should also make an effort to drink more water. A regimen of four to eight glasses a day—to be taken even if one does not feel thirsty—should be followed. Observing these simple, well known, effective principles can appreciably reduce the need for laxatives. Unfortunately many patients seem to prefer to resort to laxatives than to follow these more natural practices. Thus the best results are found in patients who have a concerned spouse able to encourage, constantly remind, and even scold as needed.

We mentioned earlier that a meal rich in protein, such as a hearty steak dinner, tends to reduce the absorption of levodopa. If levodopa is taken after such a meal, it is poorly absorbed and the therapeutic effect may be diminished. Some dietitians recommend that patients avoid excessive protein intake and limit themselves to the recommended dietary allowance of 56 grams per day for men or 46 grams for women. This is a very small amount of protein—less than that found in an ordinary one-quarter pound hamburger.

The tendency of protein to interfere with levodopa therapy suggests that low-protein diets might be useful. In fact such diets have repeatedly been studied as possible adjuncts to levodopa therapy. The results are clear: Levodopa is better absorbed on a low-protein diet—so much so that symptoms of overdosage may occur if the dose is not reduced. A smaller dose yields the same blood level and the same results when the patient is on a low-protein diet as a larger dose when the patient is on a normal diet. Unfortunately the results are otherwise similar. There seems to be no definite advantage in the low-protein diet. Moreover, it is difficult to make very low-protein diets palatable. Patients soon tire of them and revert to their customary eating habits. Dr. Jonathan Pincus of Georgetown University Medical School in Washington, D.C., has advocated a diet confining protein to the evening meal for patients with fluctuations in their response to levodopa treatment. The diet does reduce "off" episodes during the day. Although some patients have found it useful, in our experience the benefits are minimal, and the patients tire of the diet after a month or two. Several low-protein prepared food products in packets and cans have been marketed recently to Parkinson patients, with the claim of providing a nutritionally balanced and tasty diet that can aid patients with motor fluctuations gain a better control of symptoms. In our experience the best course is to adjust the dosage to the patient's customary diet, but then the diet should be consistent. Meals should be at regular times. Gastronomic excesses should be avoided.

There is no reason to forbid the use of alcoholic beverages in normal amounts. Those who are accustomed to having a glass of wine at dinner need not abandon this custom. Patients who enjoy a glass of beer or a cocktail in the evening or at a social occasion need not be deprived of this pleasure. Moderation and common sense are the watchwords here. Excesses should be carefully avoided.

Alcoholism seems to be very rare among Parkinson patients. There seems to be something about Parkinson's disease that protects against this all too common scourge. The reason is not known.

In this day of popular dietary foods, "megavitamins," "natural" foods, and health food stores, a few words about these foods in respect to parkinsonism seem in order. Generally there is no reason the Parkinson patient may not partake of these currently popular dietary fads if he or she so desires. However, there should be no hope that such foods or megavitamins can influence the disease. Some may be "good" in the sense that they are nutritious and thus "good" for anybody, but not specifically for people with Parkinson's disease.

Vitamins are substances required by the body in minute, or trace, amounts. Deficiency of the known vitamins can cause serious disturbances. Specific deficiency diseases are known for each vitamin: Scurvy results from vitamin C deficiency, beriberi from vitamin B_1 deficiency, rickets from vitamin D deficiency, and so on. If the Parkinson patient has no deficiency and eats a normal diet, taking supplemental vitamins is useless. Contrary to popular belief vitamins do not supply "pep" or energy or strength. They are taken as a sort of insurance against some possible deficiency due to poor eating habits. It is probably a good idea for older persons generally to take a multiple vitamin tablet daily, especially since the elderly often eat poorly. There is nothing specific about Parkinson patients that makes them susceptible to vitamin deficiencies. However, there is an interesting story about vitamin B_6 (pyridoxine) and parkinsonism that we might do well to review briefly.

THE PYRIDOXINE STORY

Vitamin B_6 (pyridoxine) was recommended for the treatment of parkinsonism shortly after it was first discovered about 1938. It proved ineffective, and in 1950 the American Medical Association's Council on Pharmacy consulted leading experts on the subject and concluded that pyridoxine had no place in the treatment of parkinsonism. However, pyridoxine is known to be essential for the optimal function of the enzyme that controls the chemical conversion of L-dopa (and levodopa) to dopamine in the body. For this reason when the deficiency of brain dopamine in Parkinson's disease was first discovered, there was renewed interest in pyridoxine. It was tried again in the treatment of parkinsonism in large doses: 1 gram per day or so, approximately 1,000 times more than the daily dose recommended for nutritional purposes. Again no effect was noted. Nevertheless, the notion that pyridoxine was good for persons with Parkinson's disease persists among some nutritionists, and accordingly they recommend that foods known to be rich in vitamin B_6 be included in the diet. These include wheat germ, bran, brewer's yeast, tomatoes, liver, and soybeans. Brewer's yeast is very rich in vitamin B_6 and has been recommended for Parkinson patients. These foods are perfectly fine for anyone to eat, and Parkinson patients may certainly eat heartily of them. However, no one has ever presented any evidence that patients eating these foods fare any better than patients who do not. Since pyridoxine, even in doses far larger than the amount available in foods, has been found ineffective in treating parkinsonism, it seems unlikely that foods rich in vitamin B_6 could be helpful.

In the early days of levodopa, research physicians added pyridoxine in the expectation that they would thereby enhance its conversion to dopamine. There seemed to be no advantage in doing so. In fact, to everyone's surprise, it proved deleterious. It was found that adding pyridoxine canceled out all the effects of levodopa. Patients doing well on levodopa who took "therapeutic" vitamins containing large amounts of pyridoxine suffered a gradual recurrence of their Parkinson symptoms within a week or two as if the levodopa were no longer working. When they stopped taking the vitamin pills, the levodopa gradually became effective again.

The reason pyridoxine has this effect on levodopa treatment is that the enzyme that converts levodopa to dopamine does its job so much faster in the presence of abnormally high amounts of vitamin B_6. It converts it all to dopamine before it can get a chance to reach the brain. Dopamine, alas, cannot enter the brain to reach the dopamine nerve cells of the substantia nigra. The drugs carbidopa and benserazide (see discussion in Chapter 7) have the opposite effect of pyridoxine: They inhibit the enzyme that converts levodopa to dopamine. Fortunately they do not enter the brain and thus affect the formation of dopamine inside the brain. They prevent pyridoxine from reversing the effect of levodopa in parkinsonism. Thus patients being treated with combined levodopa/carbidopa (Sinemet) or levodopa/benserazide (Madopar) can eat anything they please and take all the vitamins they wish without risking "pyridoxine reversal." However, a word of caution is in order. The protection against pyridoxine reversal may not always be complete. Thus it would still be wise to avoid "therapeutic doses" or "megadoses" of vitamins, unless they are really necessary and prescribed by a physician; the dose of vitamin B_6 should be less than 50 mg a day. Fortunately there are very few conditions that require treatment with large doses of vitamin B_6.

VITAMIN C

Vitamin C (ascorbic acid) has enjoyed a popular reputation as a preventive and treatment for the common cold ever since Professor Linus Pauling claimed it was effective in preventing colds. Very large (mega) doses have been used: 0.5- or 1.0-gram tablets one to several times daily. Whether or not vitamin C is effective in preventing colds need not concern us here. There seems to be no reason Parkinson patients may not take vitamin C in any reasonable dose. It might be used, for example, to acidify the urine in cases of bladder infection.

VITAMIN E

Vitamin E (alpha-tocopherol) has been widely promoted as being helpful in an immense variety of conditions. The large number of areas in which it has been claimed to be effective suggests that it is not effective in any. It was once widely used to relieve painful leg cramps, especially those occurring in sleep (nocturnal cramps). We have given it to Parkinson patients complaining of leg cramps, but it did not seem helpful in any. The patients sometimes thought it helped but ceased using it after awhile. Some complained it made them drowsy and tired.

For theoretical reasons, it was suggested many years ago, vitamin E may retard aging and the progression of Parkinson's disease and Alzheimer's disease. It was speculated that oxygen ions, or "radicals," played a role in these various diseases. Conclusive evidence that such is the case has been difficult to obtain. A national collaborative study called the DATATOP (Deprenyl and Tocopherol Antioxidant Therapy of Parkinsonism) study has objectively tested the possibility that vitamin E might retard the normal progression of Parkinson's disease (also see discussion in Chapter 5). High doses—2000 international units (IU) per day—were used in the study. The results did not show any effect on the signs and symptoms of Parkinson's disease. There is no evidence that vitamin E has any value in ameliorating the symptoms of Parkinson's disease or slowing the disease progression.

Vitamin E deficiency has been found to be the cause of deterioration of peripheral nerves seen in patients with chronic intestinal malabsorption or an inherited abnormality of vitamin E metabolism. The symptoms include weakness or diminished sensation in the legs and unsteadiness in walking, but nothing resembling parkinsonism. In these patients the blood level of vitamin E is very low.

So far as we know, vitamin E in reasonable doses is harmless, and there seems little reason to object to anyone using it who believes there is some benefit in it. The recommended dose is one 400-IU tablet daily.

VITAMIN B$_{12}$

Injections of vitamin B$_{12}$ (cyanocobalamin) were formerly sometimes administered by physicians as a sort of "tonic." Many patients claimed that it made them feel stronger. Physicians may give it in the hope of relieving the sense of weakness or fatigue that is so common a complaint in Parkinson patients. However, there is no known reason or clear evidence that vitamin B$_{12}$ injections are indeed helpful in dealing with these symptoms.

Deficiency in vitamin B$_{12}$ results in a particular kind of anemia, termed *pernicious anemia*. Patients with this disorder have an inability to absorb vitamin B$_{12}$ from the diet. If vitamin B$_{12}$ deficiency is suspected, tests can be done to determine if in fact there is a deficiency. The amount in the blood can be measured. If a deficiency is found, its cause should be determined by appropriate tests, and treatment with vitamin B$_{12}$ instituted. Otherwise there is no recognized justification for vitamin B$_{12}$ treatment in Parkinson patients.

MINERALS

Due to the tendency for bones to lose their calcium content gradually over the years, many physicians and nutritionists recommend supplemental mineral intake for the middle-aged and elderly. There is no evidence that such calcium ingestion really changes the gradual thinning of bones with age. However, within reasonable doses, it does no harm.

Similarly some iron solutions are often recommended, especially to menstruating women, to counter the loss of iron in menstrual blood. Iron deficiency leads to anemia, but in the absence of iron deficiency supplemental iron is useless. Iron deficiency anemia should be treated with large doses of iron, much larger than the amount in the usual vitamin tablet "fortified" with iron. In any event iron has no therapeutic effect in parkinsonism and does not relieve the sense of fatigue or weakness, unless there is indeed an iron deficiency anemia. The physician can easily determine with a blood count whether the patient is anemic, and the amount of iron in the body can be determined by sending a tube of blood to the laboratory to measure its iron content. If iron deficiency is present, the doctor can treat it appropriately. If not, there is no need to take iron or iron-fortified vitamins. Iron, incidentally, tends to increase constipation.

Sodium chloride, the mineral sprinkled on food as common table salt, may be helpful in combating the low blood pressure some patients have on levodopa therapy. The doctor should prescribe the amount of salt. Usually 1 or 2 grams per day does the trick. This is much more of course than can be obtained by salting food heavily. Salt tablets in 0.5- and 1-gram sizes are usually readily available in drug and grocery stores, especially during the summer. There are, however, potential medical complications of excessive salt intake. It may exacerbate high blood pressure, chronic congestive heart failure, and so on. Thus older persons should let their doctor decide if they need to take salt tablets.

AMINO ACID SUPPLEMENTS

The amino acid L-tryptophan was studied some years ago as a treatment for depression. Good evidence accumulated that in large doses (10 to 15 grams per day) it can indeed relieve the common depression, or "involutional melancholia," of middle age. The dose required is considerably larger than the amount one could get by dietary manipulation. Purified L-tryptophan has been sold in health food stores as a "natural" sedative and tranquilizer, but used in these small doses, it has no definite effect.

L-Tryptophan is a naturally occurring amino acid and is a precursor of the chemical messenger serotonin in much the same way that levodopa is the precursor of dopamine. Both dopamine and serotonin are present in the corpus striatum in substantial amounts. The relationships between these two important chemical messengers in the brain is not yet fully understood, but there is some evidence of antagonism. Large doses of L-tryptophan have been reported to exacerbate parkinsonism especially when combined with pyridoxine. L-Tryptophan has also been reported to diminish the severity of chorea, a condition that is in many ways the opposite of parkinsonism. Some clinicians advocated giving L-tryptophan to patients receiving levodopa to counter the side effects of the latter. However, we have found that, even given in very large doses to Parkinson patients on levodopa therapy, it produced no effect whatever on the parkinsonian state itself or on the side effects of levodopa.

It had been reported in various lay publications that L-tryptophan was beneficial for tremor. Some patients therefore obtained the amino acid at their local health food store and have taken it on their own. It is quite possible the L-tryptophan may be helpful in certain kinds of tremor, such as the severe tremulousness known as *action myoclonus*, but it is not helpful in parkinsonism.

In late 1989 the Centers for Disease Control of the U.S. Public Health Service officially recognized an epidemic of a strange malady in persons taking L-tryptophan; it was called the "eosinophilia–myalgia syndrome." Muscle aches and pains, weakness, and fatigue were the main symptoms. Cough, difficulty in breathing, skin rash, and swelling of the ankles also occurred in some cases. A marked increase in the number of "eosinophil cells" in the blood was found. These are a type of white blood cell that typically increases in allergic reactions. The mechanism of this toxic reaction was never clarified, but an impurity was suspected. L-tryptophan was withdrawn from the market in the United States.

CHOLINE AND LECITHIN

Dopamine is not the only chemical messenger affected by the ingestion of its precursor. For example, the amount of acetylcholine formed in the brain can be increased by feeding its precursor choline. Supplementing the diet with large amounts of choline chloride (10 to 15 grams daily) can suppress the involuntary movements in certain types of chorea. Choline can at least partially and transiently correct impairment of recent memory in some patients afflicted with senile mental deterioration or with Alzheimer's disease.

For several years many people obtained choline in the form of choline tartrate at health food stores or over the counter at drug stores and pharmacies in the hope of improving their mental function. There is no evidence choline can actually do so in the doses used. There is a good reason for being cautious about the use of choline in Parkinson patients. In view of the reciprocal, seesaw relationship between dopamine and acetylcholine (see discussion in Chapter 5), one might expect that increasing the formation of acetylcholine in the brain would exacerbate the parkinsonian state. And in fact it does just that! Therefore we do not advise patients to take choline. Fortunately this fad seems to have passed.

12

Common Sense About Exercise

Physical activity in amounts commensurate with one's ability and strength can make an important contribution to health and well-being. Activity is necessary to maintain the body's musculature. Unused muscles quickly atrophy.

Similarly joints need to move through their normal range of motion every day. A joint that is not used soon becomes stiff and eventually suffers a permanent loss of function. The surrounding tissues become firm and fibrotic. The joint can ultimately become frozen in a fixed posture. The patient is then said to have a *contracture* of that joint. Thus constant activity is essential to keep our musculoskeletal system with its muscles, bones, and joints functioning properly. Exercise also improves the heart and the circulation. Increased breathing during physical activity improves aeration of the lungs. The urinary tract, including the kidneys, ureters, and bladder, functions better in the upright position and is thus benefited when the individual rises and moves about. It is a common observation that physically active people have less trouble with constipation than those who lead sedentary lives. Finally physical activity has a good effect on the mind. It is relaxing, calming, and often provides a welcome change of ideas. A sense of satisfaction and well-being is a common experience following exercise.

These obvious truisms merit repetition here because, alas, Parkinson patients tend gradually to withdraw from their usual activities. For various reasons they seem to do less and less as time goes on and eventually retire to a sedentary existence if a conscious effort is not made to continue normal activities. They seem to suffer an inertia that is probably an expression of the bradykinesia of Parkinson's disease (described in greater detail in Chapter 3). To combat this tendency, it is a good idea to follow a regular routine to assure a reasonable amount of physical activity every day. Whatever the activity, it should be done daily, regularly, and in moderation. Sudden bursts of frenetic activity separated by long periods of indolence are to be deplored. A regular and constant level of activity is best. If this can be done without even thinking about it, if the patient's life style includes a regular and moderate amount of physical activity, that is all to the good. The specific nature of the activity is not important. We are not discussing physical activity as a treatment but as a means of maintaining a degree of physical fitness.

No amount of physical activity or specific type of exercise can alter the basic disease process in the nervous system. However, a patient who remains physically fit is better able to cope with the various symptoms of Parkinson's disease as the years go by. It is a matter of common experience that patients who keep physically fit fare better in the long run than patients who do not.

Some patients are fortunate in having an occupation that involves some measure of physical activity. We know a horticulturist with Parkinson's disease who retired at the usual age of 65 years. He was able to remain active in his work after retirement, working as a consultant and maintaining his own large garden and raising new rhododendron hybrids. The physical activity involved in his work provided him with an excellent quality of exercise. This man was also very fortunate in being able to continue after retirement the work he had known and loved most of his life. Some patients have a hobby or avocation that similarly entails some appreciable amount of good physical activity: fishing, hiking, rock collecting, etc. They should by all means continue these activities. How much and how often they can do so is unfortunately often limited by weather, opportunity, and the seasonal nature of some of these activities. One of our patients learned to be an amateur glider pilot shortly before the first symptoms of Parkinson's disease developed. He was able to continue this hobby for a number of years. Ultimately he had to give up gliding because of disease progression, but in the meantime he had derived pleasure and satisfaction from it, as well as some excellent physical activity. Many patients obtain perfectly good exercise through the pursuit of less dramatic but equally satisfying activities such as tending their gardens, doing light carpentry and masonry, or other yard work around the house.

Obviously those patients who are able to cultivate an interest in something that keeps both mind and body active are very fortunate. We wish it were possible for more patients to develop such interests. There are so many opportunities for leisure activities today it is a tragedy that more patients seem unable to participate. Unfortunately most patients have to carry out some program of exercise as a routine chore. It would be much better if it were fun to do, but exercise is sufficiently important that patients should faithfully do some every day as a duty to themselves, even if it seems dull. It is a good idea for many patients to have someone else monitor the performance of their daily exercise routine whatever it may be. The patient's wife or husband, relative, or friend should see to it that it is done. The patient may need to be reminded. The monitor should be prepared to urge, coax, and even insist that the exercise be done. Spouses naturally resent the role of drill sergeant, but it is a fact that patients whose devoted spouses see to it that some daily physical activity is done and done properly, fare much better than those who are allowed to lapse into sedentary and inactive lives, slumped all day before a television set.

Exercise machines, stationary bicycles, rowing machines, and similar devices are very popular, and many patients use them happily and with benefit. However, there is nothing specific about this type of indoor exercise. It is useful when one cannot get more natural exercise. All that is really necessary is to put every muscle and joint through its normal range of motion a few times every day. The exercise need not be intensive or of long duration. It should not be pushed to the point of exhaustion or discomfort.

Walking is an excellent and moderate exercise. The speed, duration, and terrain can be varied to suit the patient's ability and strength. It is not tiring. Indeed, many patients find walking refreshing and relaxing. It is a convenient form of exercise that can be done equally well in the city, suburbs, or country. One can make a point of walking every day in the course of doing certain errands, for example, walking to the corner store to get the newspaper every day. The return walk can be by a circuitous route, perhaps a different one now and then to give some variety. Walking a mile a day is a reasonable and quite common goal. Some patients find this too mild an exercise. Others can walk considerable distances in the pursuit of some hobby. One patient for many years walked throughout the city of New York to satisfy his interest in historical buildings. Another walked extensively through the fields and woodlands of New Jersey, collecting and studying wild flowers. He became something of an expert on the wild flowers of that area. Another patient, an admitted "physical fitness nut" jogs every morning. He had been jogging for years before Parkinson's disease developed, and continued this habit. More than 15 years later, he still jogs a mile every morning. This vigorous exercise has no doubt greatly benefited him, but we would not routinely recommend jogging to all patients and would not advise it for older patients who are not accustomed to it.

Swimming is also an excellent exercise. Patients who were good swimmers in earlier years may find this a satisfying activity to pursue. Of course they need regular access to a suitable facility, preferably one available throughout the year. Swimming must be done under adequate supervision. Patients subject to recurrent episodes of bradykinesia may suddenly find themselves in serious trouble in the water should they suddenly freeze and be unable to function. Patients with significant disturbances of equilibrium and walking should also avoid water activities. They are likely to have difficulties wading in shallow water and often also have trouble controlling their bodies when swimming in deep water. They may need to be rescued by a lifeguard. It is a cardinal rule of water safety that no one should swim alone. The best of swimmers heed this rule for they realize that they are not immune to having a cramp or some other accident in the water. Certainly Parkinson patients cannot ignore this rule.

Patients who have athletic skills in various sports such as tennis, golf, or squash should continue these activities. Of course they can rarely be done on a daily basis and thus cannot be the only activity used for exercise. However, the pursuit of a learned skill is an excellent way to get healthful exercise. Learned or acquired skills are apt to be less affected by parkinsonism than automatic instinctive activities such as walking. Thus patients who are able to continue a sport of this type requiring considerable motor skill can enjoy a quality of exercise that would otherwise be difficult if not impossible for them to obtain in other activities. Experienced mountain climbers, water skiers, acrobats, or what-have-you should by all means continue their activities within reason and safely within their capabilities and the limitations imposed by parkinsonism.

CALISTHENICS

Some persons have cultivated the habit of doing calisthenic exercises as a daily ritual, usually on arising in the morning or on retiring in the evening. This excellent habit should certainly be continued by those with Parkinson's disease. Of course age and general health are important factors that determine which exercises can be done. Obviously push-ups, skipping rope, or jogging are too strenuous for elderly persons or those with heart disease or arthritis. Those with a diminished exercise tolerance may do simpler exercises, however, such as bicycling motions with the legs, circling movements with the arms, bending movements, and perhaps even squatting and sitting-up exercises. These various movements may be described as active range-of-motion exercises. They assure that every large joint and its related muscles are put through their full range of motion. Repeated 5 to 10 times or more in a systematic way, these exercises can be very helpful in maintaining physical fitness.

We hesitate to recommend any specific set of exercises for so diverse a group of people as the population of Parkinson patients who may come across these pages. However, for the average patient 50 to 70 years of age whose symptoms are reasonably well controlled by proper medical treatment, perhaps the following simple calisthenics may be suggested. Many patients find these too mild and wish to do more. Others may find one or two of these exercises too strenuous or difficult. The patient should consult a physician before embarking on these exercises to be sure there are no medical reasons for not doing them. In any case these are offered simply to illustrate the type of exercises that many patients find helpful. Usually they are done in the morning on first arising but can of course be done at any time. No exercise should be continued that causes pain or discomfort or seems too difficult.

1. While lying flat on your back in bed, slowly lift one leg, knee bent, as high as you can; then straighten the leg until the toes point to the ceiling. Hold this position for 30 to 60 seconds, then slowly lower the leg to the surface of the bed. Repeat 5 to 10 times, first with one leg, then with the other.
2. Lying flat on your back, bend your head slowly to the right to bring the ear close to the shoulder; then slowly bend to the left in the same manner. Repeat 10 times in each direction.
3. Still lying flat on your back, clasp your hands behind your head and try to sit up. Repeat 5 times. (This may be too difficult for some patients.)
4. Turn over to lie on your stomach. Place your hands behind your back; then lift the head, look up to the ceiling, and try to lift the chest off the surface of the bed. Now turn your head to the right and to the left, 5 times in each direction.
5. Sit up on the side of the bed, feet on the floor, and place hands on hips. Lean forward as far as possible, then lean backward but do not fall back onto the bed; sit up straight, then lean first to the left, then to the right until the elbows touch the surface of the bed. Repeat 5 to 10 times.

6. Stand up straight with hands on hips, head held high, shoulders back, and chest thrown forward. March in place 20 steps. Be sure to raise the knees up high and count out loud.
7. Stand erect, raise arms out to side, bringing hands to the level of the shoulders. Then raise arms and bring hands together over your head. Slowly lower arms to the horizontal, pulling the shoulders as far back as possible. Finally lower arms to the side. Repeat 5 times.
8. Stand erect, then bend forward from the hips in a relaxed manner. Allow the arms to fall downward, your hands hanging limply, fingers pointing to the floor. Do not force yourself to touch your toes with your fingers. This usually happens easily after you have done this exercise a number of times. Stand up straight. Repeat 10 times.

Gentle, sensible exercises for older persons are illustrated in various videotapes. One we especially like is the program prepared by Angela Lansbury, the well-known actress and star of the television serial "Murder She Wrote." Many of her exercises should be useful to Parkinson patients.

THERAPEUTIC EXERCISES

We have been discussing activities and exercises of a general nature, useful to anyone—not only patients with Parkinson's disease—interested in maintaining physical fitness. There are, however, certain types of exercises that may be done with the aim of helping patients deal with specific Parkinson symptoms such as stooped posture, the tendency to shuffle on walking, trouble getting up out of deep chairs, or the various other difficulties these patients have when carrying out ordinary tasks of daily life. Ideally therapeutic exercises should be prescribed by a physiatrist, a physician trained in the medical specialty of physical medicine and rehabilitation, and should be performed by the patient under the supervision of a physical therapy nurse or technician, usually called a physical therapist. Most community hospitals have a department of physical medicine and rehabilitation where physical therapy can be obtained on a doctor's referral. Physical therapists may also provide treatment in freestanding facilities on a doctor's prescription. For those who are home-bound, periodic visits by a physical therapist to instruct the patient in the exercises can be very helpful. The patient, however, must do the exercises at home alone every day, preferably under the watchful eye of his or her spouse, relative, or friend. Often the patient needs some assistance to perform certain exercises. At the next visit the therapist can check the progress achieved, see that the patient is still doing the exercises properly, and modify the exercises or suggest new ones as needed. The therapist can reinforce the patient's performance by repeating the instruction and supervising the actual performance of the exercises.

The best exercises are *active* exercises done by the patient. The role of the therapist visiting the patient at home is mainly to see that the patient knows how to do the exercises and that an appropriate program of activities is being done. If necessary, the therapist can also administer passive range-of-motion and stretch exercises that the patient cannot do alone. However, such exercises must be done daily. It is not practicable to have a therapist visit the home daily, so the spouse or someone else must learn to do this type of physical treatment if it is needed. The therapist can teach the technique.

The following exercises are frequently recommended for specific problems. These are only a few examples. The therapist can teach additional ones or modify these to meet the special needs and circumstances of each patient. They should be done regularly, every day. They may help only for a short time after each performance, but a cumulative beneficial effect can usually be discerned after weeks of diligently practicing them every day.

FIG. 11. Exercise for stooped posture.

Exercises for Stooped Posture

1. Back up against a wall, making sure that heels, shoulders, and the back of the head all touch the wall. Stand in this position for 1 minute, then walk—or better yet—march across the room stepping high, and return to the wall. Turn about and back up against the wall again. Note how much you have slumped forward during your march across the room and back. Repeat the entire exercise 5 times in the morning and again 5 times in the evening (Fig. 11).
2. Stand facing the wall, raise your hands as high as possible, and lean forward, placing the palms of your hands on the wall. Slowly push your hands up the wall as far as you can reach, arching your neck and spine backward a little and stretching upward. Repeat 5 times twice a day.

FIG. 12. Exercise for shuffling and festination.

Exercises for Shuffling and Festination

1. Practice walking or marching with high steps. Count a military-type marching cadence and keep time: "hup, two, three, four, left, right, left, right," and so on. Listen to the sounds of your feet striking the floor to get the rhythm.
2. If there is still difficulty raising the feet, place a series of books, magazines, wood sticks, or other objects of similar size in a line across the room about one step apart. Step over these objects while marching across the room (Fig. 12).
3. When freezing occurs and the feet feel glued to the floor, practice rocking from side to side, swinging the arms, and counting a marching cadence out loud. If this fails, stop a moment, think about something else, and then try again. Marching in place for a few steps may also help to break through the "block."

Exercise for Sitting and Rising from Chairs

If you have particular trouble getting up out of chairs, practice sitting down and rising. Use a simple straight-back chair. Study carefully the mechanics of sitting

FIG. 13. Exercise for sitting and rising from chairs.

down and getting up out of a chair. To get up, slide forward on the seat, lean forward from the hips so that the trunk is inclined forward approximately 45 degrees, position your feet with one foot under the edge of the seat and the other a half step forward, and then place your hands on the sides of the seat near the front legs of the chair. Now push and step forward in one continuous smooth motion (Fig. 13). If necessary, count to yourself: "one, two, three, GO!" If you fail on the first attempt, rest a moment and try again. Try to get up suddenly before the Parkinson bradykinesia has a chance to block the movement.

To sit down, approach the chair briskly, turn about, then bend the trunk forward 45 degrees and sink down S L O W L Y onto the seat. Be careful to turn a sufficient amount to assure that you end up properly centered on the seat. Try not to fall or slump into the chair. For practice sit and rise 5 to 10 times. Pay careful attention to each step in the sequence. A common failing is to sit down before turning about fully, with the result that the patient sits on one half of the chair or misses the chair entirely and ends up on the floor. Proper footwork is the key. It helps if one foot is slightly behind the other and directly under the seat.

Speech Exercises

Patients whose speech is difficult for others to understand may benefit from practicing singing and reading aloud. Read the headlines from the daily newspaper, exaggerating the enunciation of each syllable. Sit before a mirror and watch the movements of the lips and tongue while reciting. Go slowly, breathe deeply, and forcefully blow out each syllable separately and loudly to practice projecting the voice. Listen carefully for each consonant and pause between the words. Recite to a measured beat marked by your hand or foot.

Patients are often not fully aware of their speech impairments. There seems to be some defect in their auditory self-monitoring. It may thus help to practice speaking into a tape recorder. Listen as you play back the phrase or newspaper headline you have just recited. Do it again, trying to correct the deficiencies you heard. By repeating this several times at one sitting you will find that it is possible to improve speech function to a considerable degree.

If speech impairment is a major problem, ask your doctor to refer you to a qualified speech therapist.

Miscellaneous

Making faces before a mirror helps to maintain the mobility of the facial muscles. Grin, frown, smile, snarl, pout, whistle, and puff out the cheeks.

If chewing and swallowing food is a problem, make an effort to chew first on one side, then on the other. Note the sound of the teeth while chewing; maintain the rhythm. Swallow small, well-chewed morsels only. Avoid the common habit of quickly swallowing half-chewed food.

SENSORY REINFORCEMENT

You may have noticed in these various exercises we have stressed the importance of sensory stimuli. Counting out loud a marching cadence, using visual cues to guide the feet, and rocking from side to side to provoke stepping are all means of enhancing the sensory stimuli with which we normally, although unconsciously, monitor motor performance in complex activities. Consciously adding strong stimuli addressed to sight, hearing, and the sense of the body's position in space serves to reinforce the normal physiological mechanisms underlying the performance of complex motor acts such as walking, talking, getting up out of a chair, and so on. This sensory reinforcement is a useful principle in physical therapy, especially in the therapy of Parkinson patients. Patients can learn to make effective use of it in many circumstances, each in his own individual manner. Many of our patients have discovered this principle by themselves. One patient controlled his drooling tendency by constantly keeping a piece of raw carrot in his mouth. Its mere presence served to stimulate an increased frequency of swallowing and thus prevented the excessive accumulation of saliva in the mouth. Another patient had nails placed in the heels of her shoes. She listened to the resulting "click clack" as she walked. She found that it made her conscious of the rhythm of her walking and prevented episodes of festination that had been troubling her gait. Many patients have discovered other similar tricks that have helped them function better.

The principle of sensory reinforcement is employed in the formal physical therapy of Parkinson patients with good effect. Walking exercises, for example, are done in a group session with a number of patients to the beat of a drum. Calisthenics are similarly done in a group to the accompaniment of music with a strong rhythmic beat.

TIPS FOR PROBLEM SITUATIONS

Patients having particular trouble with their equilibrium during walking should have more formal gait-training exercises under the supervision of a physical therapist, preferably in a properly equipped physical medicine facility. Several suggestions have often proved helpful. First, consider shoes. If the patient shuffles, he or she will probably do better in shoes with leather or hard-composition soles. Shoes with rubber soles, especially crepe rubber, may be more comfortable to wear but cannot easily slide on most surfaces. Consequently shuffling with a soft rubber sole is likely to make the foot stick to one spot, possibly causing loss of balance and a fall.

Patients who tend to step backward a few steps involuntarily (retropulsion)— and are thus subject to falling backward—may benefit from wearing shoes with heels. A heel lift inside the shoe may also help. Slippers with flat heels or no heels tend to increase the tendency to retropulsion. On the other hand patients who have more difficulty with propulsion (falling forward) may do better on low or flat heels. Scatter rugs and mats are an additional hazard for patients who shuffle. It may be a wise precaution to remove them from the home. Door sills may also be a problem, since freezing and festination indoors occur particularly at doorways. If necessary, door sills can easily be removed by a carpenter.

Patients who have trouble getting out of chairs should learn to avoid deep, upholstered chairs, especially those with low seats and soft cushions. Try to choose instead straight-back wood chairs, preferably with arm rests, such as the traditional "captain's chair." Remember the exercise described above for getting out of chairs. Be sure to move forward to the edge of the seat, position the feet for proper leverage, and push up with both hands, leaning forward as you get up. If the patient needs help getting up from a chair, merely holding his or her hand and providing slight support may suffice. The mere contact of the hand seems to provide a necessary reference point. The sensation seems more important than the actual force or support provided. If that does not do the trick, the patient's companion may then place one hand on the patient's head and push forward gently but firmly. As the patient then tries again to get up, he or she may exert considerable back pressure against the companion's hand; however, the patient nearly always can rise briskly. Very little pressure is usually required. One can often help patients who have great difficulty in getting up with the pressure of one finger. It is much easier to help them in this way than standing in front and pulling up and forward with the hands. That may sometimes be needed, but one must be careful. Patients can be pulled up to standing only to fall on top of their helpers, with both ending up on the floor.

Reclining chairs can be obtained with a spring-loaded, lever-actuated or motor-driven seat that pushes the patient up and forward on arising. Some patients find these chairs very helpful, but those with poor equilibrium may have difficulty. As they are pushed up and forward, they must be able to step forward. Patients who have difficulty standing and stepping forward may instead fall forward. We strongly advise a patient contemplating the purchase of such a chair to try it out first and be sure that it is actually helpful.

A simpler trick is to have the rear legs of the patient's favorite chair raised about 2 inches (5 or 6 centimeters) with blocks or a crossbeam. This gives the seat a slight forward tilt that makes it easier for the patient to get up and yet does not make the chair less comfortable.

A cane provides less support to the Parkinson patient with a walking problem than might be expected. Even walkers are often disappointing. The patient with poor balance and subject to episodes of retropulsion simply falls backward—cane, walker, and all. Canes can be helpful to the patient with propulsion, and many patients do learn to use them effectively. Four-legged canes are helpful to patients with poor equilibrium. There are many varieties of canes and walking aids, and the patient should be trained in their proper use by a physical therapist. The therapist can also ascertain what type of device will be most helpful. Many patients use the cane not for support but as a guide, placing it on the floor slightly ahead of the foot about to step forward. This tells the brain where to put the foot down for the next step. It provides "sensory reinforcement," just as counting a cadence or walking over markers on the floor does.

Patients with severely impaired walking and poor equilibrium who are subject to frequent falls may nevertheless have very good stepping movements; they may be able to walk well, providing they are accompanied by someone who can catch them in time to prevent a fall. Such patients should have a brief daily walk with someone in attendance as a form of exercise.

Attention to the disposition of furniture around the house helps prevent injuries in case of falls. There should be an adequate rail on stairways. Hand bars on the wall near the bathtub and toilet should be installed. The toilet seat can be raised an inch or two with blocks. A chair can be placed in the shower stall or in the bathtub to render bathing easier and safer. Rubber bath mats should help reduce the chance of falls in the bathroom.

Those patients who have difficulty dressing, buttoning clothes, tying shoes, etc. due to lack of fine control of finger movements may benefit from several modifications of their clothing. Where possible, zippers or patches of adhesive cloth can be used instead of buttons. Polo shirts or T-shirts may be used in place of front-buttoned shirts. Shoelaces may be replaced by elastic laces that do not need to be tied or untied. Loafers or similar slip-on shoes without laces may be even more comfortable.

REHABILITATION SERVICES

Most patients need only practice a simple regimen of exercises on their own or with the help of their families to maintain a normal amount of physical activity. Some patients in addition may benefit from the occasional assistance of a physiatrist and a program of physical therapy with exercises along the lines of those just discussed. A small number of more severely affected patients who have problems carrying out the ordinary activities of daily life may need more intensive physical therapy to prevent invalidism. If the symptoms of Parkinson's disease become so severe, despite good medical treatment, that the patient can no longer manage to live independently at home, whether alone or with his or her family, then perhaps admission to a hospital or to a special rehabilitation unit for a thorough evaluation and a more intensive course of physical therapy may be indicated.

A patient who has deteriorated more rapidly than expected deserves a complete medical evaluation to make sure that some other disease process is not complicating the scene. The first indication that something else is going on—an ulcer, a kidney infection, a cancer, or some other serious illness—may be a patient's unexpectedly rapid decline over a period of months after doing quite well in controlling the symptoms of Parkinson's disease. If something is found, it may be possible to correct it and restore the patient to his or her former health. Perhaps nothing serious will be found, but revision of treatment in a hospital setting may prove beneficial. Intensive physical therapy while in the hospital is usually an important part of such treatment.

In the hospital physical therapy can be given daily, and every aspect of the patient's performance of daily living activities can be reviewed. Special training can then be given to teach the patient ways of overcoming the disabilities imposed by parkinsonism, and to eat, dress, bathe, comb, brush, and do the numerous ordinary tasks of daily life. In addition, intensive physical therapy can improve the patient's gait, posture, equilibrium, and performance of various motor acts.

When the patient returns home, every effort should be made to continue some physical therapy to maintain the benefits gained in the hospital for as long as possible. The program of exercises must be carried out daily. A visit every week or two to the physical medicine department at the hospital serves to check progress and review the home exercise program. If necessary, arrangements can often be made to have a physical therapist visit the patient at home. The therapist may be able to make useful recommendations regarding the patient's life at home, the installation of hand rails and grab bars, and the use of various self-help devices. It may also be advisable to obtain some help at home. A part-time attendant or "home health aide" may be necessary to help the patient and family cope with the invalidism of advanced Parkinson's disease. The goal is to try to keep the patient at home and as independent as possible for as long as possible. The periodic visits of the visiting nurse service, if there is one in the area, may be very helpful. The visiting nurse can give valuable advice, help make arrangements for physical therapy, transportation to the doctor's office or clinic, and provide home health aids and other medical social services.

Unfortunately it is often difficult to convince the "third party" organizations such as the Medicare carriers, Medicaid, and other health insurers to pay for physical therapy and other services at home for patients with chronic diseases. They do not seem to mind paying for such care to a patient recovering from a fracture or a stroke who needs therapy for only a limited time, but they are very reluctant to commit their funds and personnel to a course of therapy that may need to be continued indefinitely. They do not seem to understand that providing limited services at home, such as a weekly visit by a physical therapist and a visiting nurse, is in the long run a great deal better for the patient and a lot less expensive than the alternative of chronic care in a nursing home.

CHRONIC CARE FACILITIES

Ultimately the patient with far-advanced Parkinson's disease may become too great a burden for the family, and at that point placement in a nursing home or chronic care hospital must be considered. Each case of course is different and must be evaluated on its individual merits. Some families are able to set up what is in effect a nursing home at home, with hospital equipment, private nurses and attendants, and so on. Most families, however, lack the resources—personal, emotional, and economic—to pursue such a demanding course. Moreover, it is not necessarily the best course for the patient. It is rarely possible to reproduce at home all the services and quality of care that are provided by the better nursing homes. For many patients rendered invalid by severe parkinsonism, a nursing home is preferable. Before making the final decision to seek nursing home placement, the patient and family will probably meet with a medical social worker.

Usually contact with a medical social worker is first made in the hospital at the request of the patient's doctor. It may be arranged through the visiting nurse service. The social worker here provides an essential service. The worker can review with the patient, the spouse, or other relative assuming responsibility for the patient's needs the available resources, doctor's recommendations, and the prognosis. Applications to suitable homes can then be initiated. The spouse or other responsible person should, if possible, visit the various facilities being considered. In most areas there is a substantial waiting period for admission to a chronic care facility. It may be 2 to 3 months or more before a vacancy is likely to open up in a desirable home. Thus the patient may have to go home for a time to await admission to the nursing home of his or her choice.

Among the things to consider in choosing a nursing home is the availability of good physical therapy. Is there a suitably equipped physical therapy facility? Are full-time physical therapists employed? Can bedside therapy be given if needed? In even the patient with the most far-advanced case of Parkinson's disease who is confined to bed and chair, physical therapy can offer much relief of discomfort and help with specific troublesome symptoms. Active and passive movement of the limbs, training in the fine art of using a wheelchair to full advantage, and ambulating with support if necessary can all make significant contributions to the patient's comfort and general well-being at this stage of the disease.

In summary exercise has a definite place in the management of Parkinson's disease at every stage in its evolution. The choice of type of activity is a highly individual matter to be decided in consultation with the treating physician. In earlier stages of the disease, informal exercise and physical activity intended to maintain physical fitness are important. The problems that arise with more severe disease can be mitigated by specific exercises. Later, more intensive physical therapy may be required. Finally even in the most advanced stages of the disease, great benefit is provided by physical therapy. Indeed it is in the later and more severe stages of the disease that physical therapy can make its greatest contribution. One final word of advice may be offered to all Parkinson patients on this general subject: Never give up any activity, never give up an inch of your independence until you absolutely must, for it is much more difficult to regain a lost activity than to hold onto it a little longer with the aid of some judicious exercise or physical therapy.

13

A Historical Perspective

Our present understanding of parkinsonism did not spring into being overnight but grew gradually over a long period of time, very slowly at first and then more and more rapidly. Most of our present knowledge was gained in the last 20 years. It has grown and changed appreciably even during the last few years. Doubtless it is changing, even as we write this passage, and will surely continue to change during the years ahead. It is thus not possible to give a final version of the truth about parkinsonism. It is not even possible to give the illusion that we can do so at this time, in the last decade of the 20th century, because our knowledge and our concepts of the brain are evolving very rapidly. For this reason, as well as for putting some concepts in perspective, it is helpful to review briefly the history of our knowledge of parkinsonism.

The modern history of parkinsonism may be said to have begun in 1817 when James Parkinson published a small monograph, *An Essay on the Shaking Palsy*. In its pages we find the first clear description of the condition we now call Parkinson's disease. The description is admittedly incomplete. Parkinson, a physician and surgeon practicing in London, had seen 6 cases over a period of some time. He was able to examine only 1 of these. It must be remembered here that the physical examination carried out by the modern medical practitioner had not yet been developed. None of the clinical techniques needed for evaluating the nervous system were then known. Neither the stethoscope nor the reflex hammer was yet in use. Moreover, the modern reader finds Parkinson's literary style quaint and archaic. Nevertheless, his account is remarkable for its accuracy and clarity of expression. In a few words he cut right to the heart of the matter. His opening chapter begins with the following terse yet comprehensive definition:

"*Shaking Palsy (Paralysis Agitans)*: Involuntary tremulous motion, with lessened muscular power, in parts not in action and even when supported; with a propensity to bend the trunk forwards, and to pass from a walking to a running pace; the senses and intellect being uninjured."

Some of the symptoms mentioned in this definition had been described long before. Indeed the ancient Greek-Roman physician Galen wrote of tremor of the hand at rest and distinguished it from a tremor occurring during movement. That is, Galen made a distinction between a resting tremor and an action tremor. It is thus tempting to believe that Galen knew of Parkinson's disease, but we cannot be certain because he does not associate the tremor with the other symptoms. Similarly, the tendency "to pass from a walking to a running pace" had also been described long before Parkinson's time. Indeed Parkinson himself referred to a description rendered by the 18th century French physician Sauvages, who had termed the abnormal gait *sclerotyrbe festinans*. On reading Sauvages' account, one feels that he had very probably seen cases of Parkinson's disease. Yet since he did not mention any other symptom, we cannot be certain. Goethe, the great German poet, noted that the innkeeper in Rembrandt's sketch "The Good Samaritan" stands in a stooped posture, holding his hands before him with the thumbs opposing the fingers as if counting coins—as patients with Parkinson's disease often do (Fig. 14). Goethe commented that the artist had been so skillful that the innkeeper's hands actually appear to tremble. One wonders if Rembrandt had intended to represent a case of Parkinson's disease, by whatever name (if any) it was known in his time. It is tempting to believe that so acute an observer as the great artist undoubtedly must have seen persons with what we now call Parkinson's disease—but again we cannot be certain.

There are other hints that Parkinson's disease has been with us a very long time. However, the possibility that James Parkinson was describing a truly new disease cannot be dismissed. A major problem is that the art of medicine was not sufficiently advanced prior to James Parkinson's time to provide much light on the subject. Very few diseases were known in their entirety. Every symptom was described as an independent entity unto itself. Medical writing was replete with descriptions of symptoms but not of entire patients.

It was only toward the end of the 18th century that combinations of symptoms came to be recognized as expressions of specific diseases that had a beginning, a particular pattern of evolution, and a termination. It was also at that time that symptom combinations came to be explained by, or at least correlated with, anatomical changes that were found on post-mortem examination. The early 19th century was a time when many of the diseases known today were first described, and a beginning was made at correlating the symptoms present in life with changes found on post-mortem study. Many of these diseases bear the names of the early medical investigator who first described them. Thus we have from the early 19th century not only Parkinson's disease but also Bright's disease, Hodgkin's disease, Bell's palsy, and so on. In many cases the names of the early describers have been dropped and more descriptive names have been used. In a few cases, however, no satisfactory term has been found, and so the eponym (the name of the physician who first wrote about the disease) remains in common use. Thus it is with Parkinson's disease.

No satisfactory descriptive term for Parkinson's disease has been found. The original term "shaking palsy" seems too vague. Its Latin translation *paralysis agitans* is no better, although it may sound more "scientific" merely because it is Latin. Diseases that were first identified from post-mortem studies are often des-

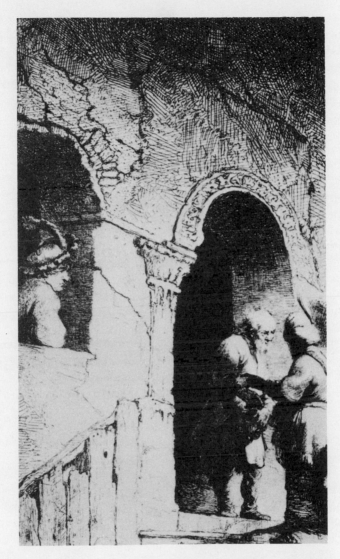

FIG. 14. The Good Samaritan in Rembrandt's famous etching. The poet Goethe thought the innkeeper seemed to have tremor of the hands. The man's appearance is suggestive of Parkinson's disease.

ignated by terms describing the essential pathological findings. Thus we have among nervous system disorders such entities as spinocerebellar degeneration, striatonigral degeneration (SND), and olivopontocerebellar atrophy (OPCA). These conditions are commonly known among neurologists by their acronyms, such as OPCA, because their names are otherwise too cumbersome to use. Following this pattern, we might describe Parkinson's disease as "substantia nigra atrophy." How-

ever, Parkinson's disease was fully recognized by its signs and symptoms long before its pathology was identified, and so the name Parkinson's disease has been
established by a long and continuous usage. There seems to be no good reason to
change the name at the present time, and it seems appropriate to commemorate
the history of our knowledge of the disorder in its name. After all, Parkinson deserves recognition for having connected the several symptoms he noted and for
having recognized that patients at "different stages of its progress" were victims
of the same disorder. This was an important contribution and a considerable accomplishment in his time.

Many other 19th century physicians contributed to our knowledge of Parkinson's disease. One especially deserving mention was Jean-Martin Charcot, a great
medical teacher and one of the founders of modern neurology. Charcot studied
patients with the shaking palsy and considerably enlarged Parkinson's description. He added the muscular rigidity, the small handwriting (micrographia), the
characteristic posturing of fingers and toes, and many other manifestations. A
scholarly man with a keen interest in history, Charcot insisted that the shaking
palsy should be named Parkinson's disease because Parkinson had been the first
to describe it and the term shaking palsy seemed inappropriate. There was, he argued, no true paralysis or palsy (as in stroke, for example) and some patients had
no tremor.

One of Charcot's students, Paul Richer, was also an artist. He is best remembered today for a textbook on human anatomy he wrote for artists (which has recently been translated into English by Robert Hale). His sketches of Charcot's patients at the Sâlpétrière hospital in Paris are classics of medical illustration and
were widely reproduced in medical textbooks of the later 19th century. One of his
sketches is shown in Fig. 15. The English neurologist, William Gowers, one of the
founders of neurology, the inventor of the ophthalmoscope, and a friend of Charcot, also described the condition in great detail. He speculated about its possible
cause and spoke of a loss of vitality of certain centers in the nervous system, a
process he termed "abiotrophy."

As a result of the work of Charcot, Gowers, and other medical teachers, Parkinson's disease became a well-recognized disorder by the late 19th century. It seems
fair to say that physicians of the 1890s were as familiar with it as physicians are
today.

Parkinson had been able only to speculate on the cause of the disease and on
the location of the disturbance in the nervous system. He expressed the hope that
"those who humanely employ post-mortem anatomical examination in detecting
the causes and nature of diseases" would be able to ascertain its "real nature" so
that "appropriate modes of relief, or even of cure," might be found.

Many physicians engaged in studying the pathology of nervous system disorders sought to find the nature of the disease as Parkinson had hoped. Their labors,
however, were for a long time unproductive, and there was much speculation regarding the site of the trouble in the brain. Some thought the problem was in the
spinal cord, and others thought it was in the muscles, but mostly no consistent ab-

FIG. 15. Sketch of patient Anne Marie Gavr . . . at the Sâlpétrière hospital in Paris, drawn by Paul Richer in 1874.

normality could be found. Parkinson's disease was thus classified for a time as a "neurosis," meaning thereby that there was no known *structural* change in the brain to explain the symptoms. In short there was an obvious disturbance of function without an apparent material cause. One can readily see on reading discussions of the disease written during the 1890s that this was a perplexing and frustrating state of affairs.

One of Charcot's students, Edouard Brissaud, suggested that the material basis of Parkinson's disease might be found in a certain small nerve center, or nucleus, in the brainstem, called the substantia nigra. Studies of this area of the brain were later made post-mortem. There was great difficulty distinguishing changes that might be due to aging, arteriosclerosis, or the disease itself. Finally a student named Tretiakoff, working on his doctoral thesis in Paris, described a number of changes in the nerve cells of the substantia nigra that are now recognized as typical of Parkinson's disease. There was a loss of the pigmented nerve cells of this nucleus, and the spherical body first noted by Frederick Lewy was present in the remaining nerve cells. His thesis was published in 1915, nearly a century after Parkinson's *An Essay on the Shaking Palsy.* These findings were not readily accepted by the medical scientists of that time. Many neurologists were skeptical that injury to so small a group of obscure nerve cells could give rise to all the varied symptoms of parkinsonism. Others thought that loss of nerve cells in other areas, especially in the corpus striatum, was a more likely cause of the symptoms. Controversy continued on this subject for many years.

The recurrent epidemics of sleeping sickness, or encephalitis lethargica, that struck during the years 1916–1926, brought great confusion to the whole subject. Rather suddenly neurologists were confronted with large numbers of relatively young patients having symptoms bearing some resemblance to those of Parkinson's disease. There were also some striking differences. The victims of this new disease were relatively young, mostly between the ages of 15 and 30, whereas previously parkinsonism under age 40 had been extremely rare. Suddenly the young Parkinson patient had become commonplace in the neurological clinics and wards of big city hospitals. These young patients had many bizarre symptoms that had never before been associated with parkinsonism.

The recognition that there could be two kinds of parkinsonism soon led to the labeling of other conditions that bore some resemblance, however remote, to Parkinson's disease as types of parkinsonism. Thus there came about the notion of arteriosclerotic parkinsonism and parkinsonism due to carbon monoxide or other chemical intoxications. The various entities became confused—so much so that during the 1930s some physicians began to suspect that all parkinsonism was due to encephalitis! A more popular view was that there was no such thing as Parkinson's disease, but that "parkinsonism" was simply a fortuitous grouping of symptoms reflecting many different diseases. With the concept of parkinsonism in such a confused state, it is not surprising that pathologists had difficulty confirming Tretiakoff's findings.

The structural changes in the brain in cases of encephalitis lethargica were studied and defined. Here too the substantia nigra was consistently found to be affected. The change was thought perhaps to be related to the Parkinson symptoms; however, instead of Lewy bodies, the remaining cells contained a dense bundle of microscopic filaments called "neurofibrillary tangles." Then a German pathologist, Dr. Rolf Hassler, studied the substantia nigra in Parkinson's disease in greater detail and confirmed the earlier findings of Tretiakoff. His work was published in 1939, but because of the disruption of World War II it received little attention for some years. After the war the noted brain pathologist, Dr. J.G. Greenfield, studied the brains of Parkinson patients at London's National Hospital for Nervous Diseases, and further confirmed the constant involvement of the substantia nigra in Parkinson's disease. Gradually, more and more brain pathologists came to agree that here was the major site of anatomical derangement in parkinsonism and that Lewy bodies were the hallmark of Parkinson's disease, whereas neurofibrillary tangles were typical of post-encephalitic parkinsonism.

The significance of the changes observed in the substantia nigra remained obscure for a long time. No one knew what the substantia nigra did or how extensive its connections were with other brain regions. Research anatomists tried to injure the substantia nigra in animals but were unable consistently to produce manifestations similar to those of human parkinsonism. There were considerable technical difficulties, and no one was quite sure how a parkinsonian cat or dog or monkey should look.

A major step forward came with the demonstration, using a new microscopic technique developed in Sweden, that the nerve cells of the substantia nigra contained the chemical substance dopamine. The new technique depended on a chemical reaction that changes dopamine into a substance that shines brightly green when placed under ultraviolet light. In the 1960s a brilliant group of young Swedish researchers, including Drs. Ungerstedt, Dahlström, Fuxe, and Anden, applied this technique to the rat brain and demonstrated whole systems of nerve cell pathways that had previously been unknown. Among these was an important system of fibers that arose from the nerve cells of the substantia nigra and went to all areas of the corpus striatum. This new discovery in the field of brain anatomy was given additional meaning by new discoveries in other areas. Biological chemists were finding that dopamine was present almost exclusively in these two regions of the brain. One researcher, Oleh Hornykiewicz, working in the medical school of the University of Vienna, measured dopamine in the brains of patients who had died with various diseases. He found a striking deficiency of dopamine in those who had parkinsonism, but not in those with other disorders. On further work he noted that the dopamine deficiency was greatest in those cases in which the pathologists found the most severe changes in the substantia nigra.

These various biochemists owed their ability to measure dopamine, adrenalin, serotonin, and related biologically active substances in brain and other tissues to the work of Dr. Julius Axelrod at the National Institutes of Health (NIH) in Bethesda, Maryland. Many of them had come to NIH to study with Dr. Axelrod. These substances occur in minute quantities in tissue admidst innumerable other similar substances. Dr. Axelrod had developed chemical techniques for separating these substances and then measuring them in extremely small samples. He thus opened an entire new field of biological chemistry. He was awarded the Nobel Prize for Physiology and Medicine in 1970 for his discovery of the enzyme, catechol-o-methyl transferase which degrades dopamine and related chemical messengers within the nervous system after they are no longer needed to transmit nerve impulses.

Related research in animals showed that when the substantia nigra was injured, dopamine disappeared from the corpus striatum on the same side. This indicated that there must be a connection from the substantia nigra to the corpus striatum and confirmed of the existence of the *nigrostriatal* pathway. This was important because these fibers could not be demonstrated by the classic methods of brain anatomy. Brain anatomists were skeptical at first, but as this sort of evidence gradually accumulated and was confirmed by scientists in other countries, the existence of the dopamine nerve cell system gained acceptance.

In the meantime a third key observation had been made by Professor Arvid Carlsson at the University of Göteborg in Sweden. In 1957 he carried out a simple experiment that clarified the way in which reserpine produced its tranquilizing effect. Reserpine is a major tranquilizer that can produce a condition closely resembling Parkinson's disease. Chemical measurements had shown that reserpine caused depletion of various substances in the brain, including noradrenaline, dopamine, and serotonin. Some thought that the tranquilizing effect was due to the depletion of serotonin. Professor Carlsson found that an injection of levodopa immediately reversed the tranquil state produced in the animals by reserpine, whereas the precursor of serotonin did not. He also measured the amount of dopamine in the brains of the animals and found that the levodopa had restored the dopamine levels to normal.

These several discoveries achieved independently in separate scientific fields gave a new meaning to the changes in the substantia nigra first found in Parkinson patients and explained the production of parkinsonism by the tranquilizing drugs. Parkinsonism could now be defined as a state of brain dopamine insufficiency. Professors Carlsson and Hornykiewicz both suggested that levodopa might be tried as a treatment for parkinsonism. These discoveries, which so greatly clarified the nature of parkinsonism, came chiefly during the decade 1957–1967. However, they represented the culmination of many decades of scientific research and thought. They could not have been achieved, say, during the 1930s or 1940s because the basic knowledge of brain chemistry was lacking. Indeed even the fundamental techniques—such as the use of radioisotopes and the analytical techniques in organic chemistry that made possible the measurement of dopamine and related substances in the brain—were unknown before 1950. Thus it is that practical advances in medical care depend on the state of science as a whole, and that so-called "pure" research in basic science having no obvious connection to practical problems leads eventually to profound new understanding of human disease and entirely new forms of treatment.

Initially levodopa was given in small doses by injection into a vein or in small doses by mouth. The first physicians to try levodopa were Dr. Walter Birkmayer of Vienna and Dr. Andre Barbeau of Montreal, Canada. Many others soon attempted the same approach. There was marked disagreement regarding the results. Some reported dramatic improvement even in severely affected patients. Others found no effect at all, and still others noted some minimal improvements but thought they might be due to psychological factors (such as the enthusiasm of the investigators) rather than to the levodopa effect. A thoughtful review of the evidence in 1965 indicated that the results were too limited to be of practical value for the treatment of Parkinson patients.

Then Dr. George Cotzias, a medical scientist working at the Brookhaven National Laboratories in Upton, New York, found that much larger doses by mouth yielded better results. He found that if he continued to administer dopa (at first he worked with a 50-50 mixture of D-dopa and L-dopa or DL-dopa) every day for weeks and months, the patients gradually became tolerant of the side effects. Nausea and vomiting gradually diminished and disappeared, so that progressively larger doses could be given. By persisting patiently, raising the dose every few days as his patients slowly developed a tolerance for dopa, Dr. Cotzias was able eventually to give doses 20 to 30 times larger than the initial dose. With very large doses (as high as 12 to 18 grams of DL-dopa per day), he obtained striking improvements in patients with typical and quite severe parkinsonism. The effects of dopa were clearly much greater than those attainable with the conventional anti-Parkinson drugs previously available.

Dr. Cotzias first reported his results with DL-dopa in 1967. Within a year they were confirmed at several other research centers. A large, carefully controlled study conducted by Drs. Yahr, Hoehn, Barrett, Schear, and Duvoisin at the Columbia–Presbyterian Medical Center in New York and similar studies carried out by Drs. Sweet and McDowell at New York Hospital, by Dr. Markham at the University of California in Los Angeles, and many others helped gain acceptance of levodopa administration as a normal treatment for Parkinson's disease.

Several thousand patients were treated under research protocols at major teaching hospitals and medical research centers throughout the United States and in many other countries. Levodopa was consistently found to be more effective in the treatment of parkinsonism than any other treatment then known. The generic name levodopa was chosen for the medical preparation of L-dopa as a drug. It was formally approved by the Food and Drug Administration (FDA) for use in treating parkinsonism in 1970.

In the quarter century since the advent of levodopa treatment, much effort has been expended to improve its action. The dopamine receptor agonists, bromocriptine (Parlodel) and pergolide (Permax), gradually found their place as drugs that improve the beneficial effects of levodopa. The later addition of selegiline (Eldepryl) (also known generically as deprenyl) provides another means of enhancing the good effects of levodopa. The demonstration that constant infusions of levodopa markedly diminish severe fluctuations of the on–off effect led to the development of slow-release, or controlled-release, formulations of levodopa in combination with carbidopa (Sinemet CR) and levodopa in combination with benserazide (Madopar HBS), which further enhance the efficacy of levodopa. These refinements and enhancements of levodopa treatment were limited but significant improvements in the treatment of parkinsonism.

THE MPTP STORY

In 1977 a young man living in Arlington, Virginia, made a fateful and unintentional discovery. An amateur chemist addicted to narcotic drugs, he satisfied his craving by synthesizing in his home laboratory a drug closely related to meperidine (Demerol). He followed a simple recipe, using easily available chemicals, outlined in a journal of medicinal chemistry. After using a hastily prepared batch of his homemade narcotic, he became acutely ill, rigid, and immobile and had to be admitted to a hospital. A physician noted the resemblance of his condition to parkinsonism and prescribed levodopa/ carbidopa (Sinemet). The young man improved but had marked on–off fluctuations.

He was referred to the clinical center of the National Institutes of Health (NIH) at Bethesda, Maryland. Drs. Sandford Markey, a chemist working in Dr. Irving Kopin's laboratory at the NIH, followed his recipe and studied the young man's chemical apparatus and glassware. He found that the reaction produced not only the narcotic drug the young man had desired but also a small amount of a by-product, especially if the reaction was run at too high a temperature. Analysis showed that the by-product was in chemical terminology, N-methylphenyl tetrahydropyridine, now widely known as MPTP.

Dr. Kopin and his colleagues found that injections of minute doses of MPTP produced a Parkinson-like condition in monkeys. An animal given even a minute dose would overnight become rigid and immobile, barely able to move very slowly, unable to eat or drink. A dose of levodopa restored the animal to normal but in an hour or so it would again become rigid and immobile, exactly as in a human patient with severe on–off fluctuations. They further found that a derivative of MPTP accumulated in the brains of these animals. On analysis the derivative proved to be a substance with the chemical name N-methylphenyl tetrahydropyridinium, referred to now by the acronym MPP$^+$.

Meanwhile, the young man continued to be severely parkinsonian, responding to treatment with on–off fluctuations. Within a year he died of a narcotic overdose. His brain was studied post-mortem, and it was found that the nerve cells of the substantia nigra had been totally destroyed. Dr. Stanley Burns, a neurologist also working in Dr. Kopin's laboratory, soon found that the nerve cells of the substantia nigra had also been destroyed in monkeys rendered parkinsonian by MPTP.

A description of the young man's unfortunate misadventure was published in 1979 by Dr. Glenn Davis, a young psychiatrist, Dr. Adrian Williams, a young neurologist, and others working with Dr. Kopin. It received little notice until several years later when several drug addicts in California appeared in an emergency room with severe parkinsonism of sudden onset. They had given themselves injections of an illicit drug purchased on the street. The resemblance of this event to that of the young man from Virginia was recognized by an alert technician in the local poison control center. A neurologist called in consultation, Dr. William Langston, obtained a sample of the illicit drug from these addicts and had it analyzed. It contained MPTP!

Dr. Langston and his colleagues canvassed the local addict population and found a total of 200 who had used the same street drug. Seven of them had obvious signs of severe parkinsonism. A number were later found to have mild degrees of parkinsonism. Several other instances of MPTP-induced parkinsonism subsequently came to light. One concerned a Danish medicinal chemist who had prepared a batch of MPTP to use as a reagent in the synthesis of new analgesic drugs. He apparently allowed the MPTP to contact his skin. He became acutely ill with a flu-like illness and became parkinsonian. His doctors thought he had developed post-encephalitic parkinsonism. Levodopa treatment proved helpful. Years later, on learning of the toxicity of MPTP, his wife realized what had actually happened. The chemist was further studied by Dr. Kopin's group at the NIH in Bethesda, Maryland. Interestingly there was no evidence that his parkinsonian condition had worsened over the intervening 9 years.

Dr. Langston read a paper describing the California drug addicts rendered parkinsonian by MPTP at the annual meeting of the American Academy of Neurology in San Diego, California, in April 1983. The striking resemblance of the MPTP-induced parkinsonism to Parkinson's disease naturally suggested that a similar substance occurring in nature or perhaps as a man-made environmental pollutant might be the cause of Parkinson's disease. Researchers throughout the world promptly began to study MPTP in the hope of finding the cause of Parkinson's disease.

Within a few years the mechanism of action of the drug was worked out. A key step was the finding that MPTP was converted to MPP^+ by the enzyme monoamine oxidase (MAO). Drugs inhibiting that enzyme prevented the formation of MPP^+. Dr. Richard Heikkila at the Robert Wood Johnson Medical School in New Brunswick, New Jersey, found that mice treated first with an inhibitor of MAO were not affected by a subsequent dose of MPTP, whereas mice receiving MPTP alone suffered destruction of the nerve cells in the substantia nigra. The same phenomenon was shown in monkeys by Drs. Langston and Ian Irwin.

These and other studies showed that the toxic agent was actually MPP^+. MPTP was merely its precursor. Researchers then tried to determine how MPP^+ worked. Dr. Solomon Snyder and his colleagues at Johns Hopkins University discovered that dopamine nerve cells avidly took up MPP^+, as if it were dopamine. Drugs that blocked the uptake of dopamine into the dopamine nerve cells could also protect animals against the toxic effects of MPTP.

Drs. William Nicklas and Ivy Vyas in New Brunswick, New Jersey, soon found that, once inside the dopamine nerve cells, MPP_+ acted on a small structure found in all living cells called the mitochondrion. All living cells contain mitochondria whose main function is to carry on the metabolism of oxygen. In a sense the mitochondria are the lungs of the cell. Not surprisingly they are essential to the life of the cell. Poison the mitochondria, and the cell instantly dies. The deadly fish poison, rotenone, is a powerful mitochondrial poison. Drs. Nicklas and Vyas found that MPP^+ acted precisely as did rotenone: Both inhibit a specific enzyme system inside the mitochondria known as "complex one," thereby interrupting cellular respiration and promptly killing the nerve cells.

The discovery that MPP^+ acted by poisoning the mitochondria in so highly specific a manner was met at first with skepticism, but eventually it was confirmed by other researchers. It then led logically to examination of the mitochondria in the brains of patients with Parkinson's disease. A group of researchers in London, including Drs. A.H.V. Schapira and John Clark (a biochemist expert on mito-

chondrial disorders) found that the mitochondrial enzyme affected by MPP⁺ and
rotenone was partially deficient in the substantia nigra of patients with Parkinson's disease. This finding has been followed up by Dr. Peter Jenner in London
and by researchers elsewhere. However, it is not clear what it means.

The structural changes caused in the brain by MPTP have been extensively studied in animals, and it has become clear that MPTP-induced parkinsonism differs
from Parkinson's disease. MPTP affects chiefly the substantia nigra. It does not
affect other brain regions that are regularly affected in Parkinson's disease. Nor
does it produce Lewy bodies. Our earlier hopes that MPTP might lead us to the
cause of Parkinson's disease have not been realized. However, it has provided a
simple, efficient way of making a laboratory animal parkinsonian and thus has
been used as a tool by researchers looking for new drug treatments for parkinsonism.

The striking resemblance of MPTP-induced parkinsonism in monkeys and humans naturally suggested at first that perhaps Parkinson's disease might be due
to a similar poison occurring in nature or perhaps as man-made pollutant in our
environment. Neurologists began searching for clues to some environmental factor among their patients. They looked for exposure to pesticides and clustering of
Parkinson's disease cases in geographical regions. Although there were some reports suggesting that persons with the disease were more likely to have lived in
rural areas than other persons or to have had greater exposure to agricultural chemicals, these reports could not be confirmed by other studies. Comparisons of the
prevalence of Parkinson's disease in different countries were attempted, but no
definite clusters or major regional differences emerged. In short no clues to an
environmental factor were found.

In retrospect we can see how the resemblance of post-encephalitic parkinsonism to Parkinson's disease earlier in this century led to the search for a virus as
the cause of Parkinson's disease. In the 1980s the MPTP experience and the resemblance of MPTP-induced parkinsonism to Parkinson's disease led to a search
for another kind of environmental agent, a toxin or chemical pollutant, as a possible cause. Yet we may also note that recent studies seeking evidence of exposure
to environmental agents have instead found that the most important risk factor is
the occurrence of Parkinson's disease in other family members. Thus, in a roundabout way, the search for the cause of Parkinson's disease has brought us to the
role of heredity.

THE LEWY BODY

To the pathologist, the hallmark of Parkinson's disease visible under the microscope is a particular abnormal structure called the Lewy (pronounced la¥-veh)
body within affected nerve cells in the substantia nigra and other areas of the brain.
Lewy bodies may also be found in certain nerve cells in the spinal cord, in the
sympathetic ganglia, and in the nerve cells in the walls of the esophagus and in-

testine! Under the microscope the Lewy body appears as a round mass about the size of a red blood cell, surrounded by a clear halo. Studied by electron microscopy, it has been found to consist of short filaments arranged randomly in a dense bundle at the center but radially like the spokes of a bicycle wheel in its outer portions. Chemical analyses using various kinds of antibodies have shown that it consists of neurofilament material.

Today nearly all neurologists and neuropathologists who study parkinsonism agree: "If there are no Lewy bodies, it isn't Parkinson's disease." Put another way, what we call Parkinson's disease has come to mean that form of parkinsonism associated with Lewy bodies. Thus when we diagnose "Parkinson's disease," we believe that Lewy bodies are present. Indeed the pathologist's diagnosis has become more reliable than our clinical diagnosis. Some patients we thought too atypical in their symptoms to diagnose as Parkinson's disease have proven to our surprise to have the typical Lewy-body changes on post-mortem study. We had to conclude that despite their atypical manifestations they really had Parkinson's disease.

INCIDENTAL LEWY BODIES

Some years ago Dr. Lysia Forno, a neuropathologist at the Veterans Hospital in Palo Alto, California, looked for Lewy bodies on post-mortem study of the brains of persons who had not had any nervous system disease in life. Her purpose was to study changes in the brain associated with aging. She found Lewy bodies in 6% of the "nonparkinsonian" brains she studied! Dr. William Gibb of the National Hospital in London similarly found Lewy bodies in 5.6% of nonparkinsonians over age 40 and in more than 11% of those over age 80! Both Drs. Forno and Gibb found these Lewy bodies in the same places they occur in patients who had symptoms of Parkinson's disease in life; the Lewy bodies were also associated with other signs of nerve cell damage in the same areas. Thus both investigators concluded that these bodies were not merely "incidental" but that the persons who had these bodies in fact had Parkinson's disease that had not produced recognizable symptoms. Had these persons lived longer, they would eventually have developed Parkinson symptoms. The numbers found by Drs. Forno and Gibb tell us that there are many more persons with presymptomatic Parkinson's disease than persons who have Parkinson's disease with symptoms, perhaps 10 to 15 times as many! .

Post-mortem studies of the brains of Parkinson patients have steadily progressed over the past quarter century. The pattern of distribution of the Lewy body throughout the nervous system has been extensively studied. Some 20 years ago they began to be found in the cerebral cortex as well as in the substantia nigra of some patients studied post-mortem. Such patients were said to have "diffuse Lewy body disease." Usually, such patients had symptoms of parkinsonism plus symptoms similar to those of Alzheimer's disease. Some, however, may have had only symptoms of the latter.

For a time diffuse Lewy-body disease was thought to be a separate disorder. But neuropathologists studying parkinsonian brains post-mortem have been finding Lewy bodies more and more frequently in the cerebral cortex. They also find them in many other regions of the nervous system, even in the spinal cord, in nerve cell plexuses nearly everywhere—including the nerve cell plexuses in the walls of the intestine and esophagus.

Dr. Kosaka working at the University of Yokohama, Japan, proposed that there was a spectrum of Lewy-body disease and identified three groups of cases: types A, B, and C. Type A cases had many Lewy bodies throughout the brain. Type C had Lewy bodies only in the substantia nigra and other brainstem nerve centers. These cases corresponded to typical Parkinson's disease. Type B was intermediate. In a series of studies of brain specimens collected by the Parkinson's Disease Society of the United Kingdom, Drs. William Gibb, Robert Hughes, and Andrew Lees found Lewy bodies in the cerebral cortex in all cases of Parkinson's disease. They were found especially in certain regions of the brain, chiefly in the temporal lobes and in a portion of the temporal lob called the hippocampus. Now pathologists regularly find Lewy bodies in the gray matter of the cerebral hemispheres in all Parkinson patients studied post-mortem. Some specimens show only a few Lewy bodies in the cerebral cortex; others show many, and all degrees in between can be found.

Recently Dr. Margery Mark at the Robert Wood Johnson Medical School in New Brunswick, New Jersey, and Dr. Dennis Dickson, a neuropathologist at Albert Einstein Medical College in New York, have shown that the whole spectrum can be found within one family! They have thus confirmed that Kosaka's types A, B, and C are variations of the same condition.

HEREDITY

The role of heredity in Parkinson's disease has received increasing attention over the past 5 years. The notion that heredity plays a role in Parkinson's disease is not new. It was first advanced over a century ago by William Gowers, the English neurologist we mentioned earlier. Many reports of families with several cases of parkinsonism were recorded in medical journals in the late 19th and early 20th century. A half century ago, a young psychiatrist, Dr. Henry Mjönes, carried out a genetic study of Parkinson's disease. He was working for an advanced degree in medicine at the University of Lund, Sweden, under the supervision of Professor Sjogren, a leading geneticist of the time. A pioneering effort, it was the first systematic genetic study of Parkinson's disease.

Dr. Mjönes identified 194 patients with definite Parkinson's disease confirmed on his examination or by examinations by other physicians recorded in medical charts. He then set out to examine all the living relatives and to look up the records of deceased relatives. He found many affected brothers, sisters, and parents and identified 9 families in which the condition had occurred in two or more generations. He concluded that Parkinson's disease was a hereditary disorder, probably due to a single gene mutation, transmitted from generation to generation to both men and women.

In his analysis Mjönes pointed out that the late age of onset of Parkinson's disease in many patients concealed its familial pattern. Since many patients do not develop symptoms of parkinsonism until their 70s or 80s, or sometimes even in their 90s—that is, at ages exceeding the average life span—he argued that some persons who carry the gene and are thus at risk for parkinsonism would not live long enough to exhibit its symptoms. Comparing the age of onset in his patients with actuarial tables of life expectancy, he calculated that only 60% of persons who carry the presumed gene mutation will develop overt signs and symptoms of the disease. He also observed that some relatives had only one or two symptoms, for example, tremor alone or tremor plus loss of facial expression. These relatives with partial parkinsonism would not ordinarily be diagnosed as having Parkinson's disease by a physician.

Mjönes argued that since they were related to a typical patient, they too had the disease and he counted them as affected. The most common of these partial manifestations was the relative who had only tremor. Mjönes' report aroused little interest at the time and his conclusions were largely ignored. Most physicians then believed that parkinsonism was not a particular disease but merely a combination of symptoms due to many different conditions, including arteriosclerosis, encephalitis, and a variety of degenerative disorders that would some day be identified. Many believed that an environmental factor, the presumed virus responsible for encephalitis, was the cause of most cases. Mjönes was also criticized for counting the relatives with partial parkinsonism as also affected. He had no evidence to justify his doing so. Post-mortem examinations of the brain had been carried out in several of his patients; but these were not helpful, for pathologists did not yet know—even in 1949—how to recognize Parkinson's disease in post-mortem brain tissue samples. Dr. Mjönes was too far ahead of his time.

The late Dr. Andre Barbeau of Montreal had also observed familial clustering of parkinsonism. He noted that some of his familial patients had relatives with essential tremor but interpreted this finding differently. He thought that there was a special form of parkinsonism related to essential tremor, calling it "essential tremor-related parkinsonism." More recently Dr. David Brooks and his colleagues at the Hammersmith Hospital in London studied a number of pairs of twins and other at-risk relatives with solitary (essential) tremor, using an imaging method called positron emission tomography (PET) (see discussion below). The PET images almost always showed abnormal uptake of fluorodopa in a pattern typical of Parkinson's disease. This finding supports Mjönes' decision to count such individuals as secondary cases of Parkinson's disease.

Dr. Barbeau had also suggested that Parkinson's disease could be the result of a combination of environment and heredity. He had found that some Parkinson patients metabolized the drug debrisoquin sulfate (an antihypertensive agent) more slowly than others. It is generally believed that these differences are genetically determined. The proportion of "slow-metabolizers" of this drug was higher in a small series of Parkinson patients than in a group of normal subjects. He also noted that there seemed to be more cases of Parkinson's disease south of the St. Lawrence River than there were to the north of it, observing that the region of higher prevalence was also the region of more intense agriculture. He combined these two observations in the idea that there was an environmental toxin that was more likely to affect slow-metabolizers of debrisoquin, who presumably would not be able to detoxify as efficiently as the supposedly more normal metabolizers did.

Dr. Barbeau's colleagues later withdrew the observation about slow- and fast-metabolizers because they found that many of the patients had taken the antihistamine diphenhydramine (Benadryl) and other drugs that influence the drug-metabolizing system. Nevertheless, the idea has continued to seem attractive. Dr. Adrian Williams and his colleagues in England have pursued this subject further and have reported other differences in liver metabolism between Parkinson patients and persons without the disease.

POSITRON EMISSION TOMOGRAPHY

Positron emission tomography (PET) is a remarkable technique for imaging metabolic activities in parts of the body in three dimensions. It is a very expensive research tool requiring a large team of scientists (nuclear physicists, radiochemists, pharmacologists, engineers, and specially trained physicians), a cyclotron, and an imaging system similar to that used in the routine CT (or CAT) scan. PET studies in the past few years have provided important insights into brain dysfunction in Parkinson's disease and have proved useful in confirming the diagnosis in borderline cases.

Essentially PET scanning is analogous to a thyroid scan. A tracer substance, to which a radioactive atom has been attached, is administered to the subject, and the accumulation of this tracer in the organ or body part under study is monitored by radiation detectors. For example, iodine is extracted from the bloodstream by the thyroid gland with such high efficiency that virtually all the iodine is concentrated in the thyroid gland. By administering a minute amount of radioactive iodine and then placing detectors over the thyroid gland to record, one can obtain an image of the gland and identify abnormalities that cannot be detected by other methods.

To assess brain dopamine systems using PET scanning, a minute amount of levodopa to which a radioactive atom of fluorine has been attached is injected into the bloodstream. This fluorinated levodopa, or fluorodopa, travels through the body and is taken up by brain dopamine nerve cells just as if it were levodopa. There it is converted to fluorodopamine in just the same way that levodopa is converted to dopamine.

The radioactive atom (fluorine 18) used in PET emits positrons as it undergoes radioactive decay. A positron is an elemental particle equal in mass to an electron but carrying a positive electrical charge—whereas electrons are negatively charged. It is extremely short-lived and travels only a few millimeters at most before colliding with an electron. Both are annihilated on impact releasing a brief burst of x-radiation consisting of two beams of x-rays going off in exactly opposite directions. This fact makes it possible to determine precisely where the collision occurred.

The patient having PET scanning is placed within a ring of radiation detectors, which record the pairs of x-rays traveling in opposite directions given off by positron–electron collisions. Each collision will thus be "seen" by a pair of detectors at opposite points on the ring. Precisely where in the brain the collision took place is calculated, using a very sophisticated system of electronic circuits linked to a powerful computer, by determining the small differences in the times at which the burst of x-rays arrives at the detectors and the precise location of the detectors relative to the patient's head. From the millions of collisions taking place, the computer can make an image of the brain in much the same way as CT scanning. The CT scanner also uses an array of detectors arranged in a series of rings. In both PET and CT scanning, these rings form a tunnel in which the patient is placed during the study.

Since fluorodopa will be concentrated very rapidly within the corpus striatum, where most of the dopamine nerve fibers are located, the PET scanner will "see" an outline of the corpus striatum. Knowing the amount of fluorodopa injected and noting the intensity of the radiation arising in the corpus striatum, one can calculate the relative amount of levodopa-uptake capacity and dopamine-storage capacity in the corpus striatum. This provides a measure of the condition of the dopamine nerve cell system. Unfortunately PET gives only a crude image, which is not sufficiently detailed to show the substantia nigra itself, where the dopamine nerve cell bodies reside.

Fluorodopa PET scanning for imaging brain dopamine systems has been used for nearly a decade now at several PET centers. Decreased capacity to take up L-dopa and form dopamine in the striatum has been shown in Parkinson patients. Impairment of brain dopamine systems has been seen even before any symptoms appeared. For example, Dr. Donald Calne and his colleagues at the Tri-University PET Centre at the University of British Columbia found evidence of severely impaired brain dopamine systems in some of Dr. Langston's drug-addicted patients exposed to MPTP, even though they had no symptoms of parkinsonism. Fluorodopa PET scanning has also proved useful in presymptomatic detection of Parkinson's disease in individuals known to be at risk for the disease—at least for research purposes. Due to its expense and limited availability, PET has been limited to research use.

14

Genetics: A Family Condition?

Most of us know the parents or grandparents we come from. But we go back and back, forever; we go back all of us to the very beginning; in our blood and bone and brain we carry the memories of thousands of beings....
(From "A Way in the World," New York: Alfred A. Knopf, 1994)
—V.S. Naipaul

The 1990s have already witnessed an important change in thinking about the cause of Parkinson's disease. Whereas most neurologists through the 1980s believed an environmental factor was likely to be responsible due to the impact of the MPTP story (see Chapter 13), opinion began to change as it was recognized that there were families in which the condition appeared in successive generations in a pattern typical of inherited disorders. These familial cases showed that the cause, at least in some patients, could be genetic. At first skeptics argued that such families were rare and that most cases were probably due to some environmental factor. Gradually more and more families were found in which multiple cases had occurred. Because some familial cases had unusual symptoms or an unusually early age of onset, the patients were initially thought to have a different condition. But on further study it has become clear that the symptoms of Parkinson's disease are much more variable than we believed and that a familial pattern can be found in a large percentage of patients. Today many centers are focusing their research on the genetic aspects of Parkinson's disease.

To some Parkinson patients and their families, this news may be unexpected and somewhat scary. That is understandable. Much attention had been directed over the past several decades to the search for clues to an environmental cause. This gave rise to hope that the whole problem would soon be solved. In retrospect it is easy to see that such hope was somewhat naive and certainly excessive. How wonderful it would have been if only Parkinson's could have been traced to some specific environmental toxin that could easily be removed or neutralized! But, alas, nature is rarely so simple or obliging. Some may fear that a genetic cause will be much more difficult to overcome.

The idea that the cause of the disease lies in our genes strikes at our very sense of being. That the cause may lie within ourselves may be difficult at first to accept. It also raises a host of new questions. These may be troubling questions. For example, will other family members—in particular, the children—someday be subject to the same illness? Could we diagnose the presence of the gene before there are any symptoms? If so, could we develop a treatment to prevent it? Since we don't presently have means of delaying or preventing the disease, who would really want to know whether he or she carried the gene mutation?

Most patients see the new genetic approach in a more positive light. They see in it the hope of an eventual cure and of far better treatments. Indeed many have written or called to tell us of their families in the hope that they can help us clarify the genetic cause of the disease. Their positive attitude is fully justified. The present state of knowledge of human genetics and the remarkable power of modern DNA molecular analysis provide the quickest and surest road to a cure and means of prevention. Geneticists have recently begun to examine multiple-case families, seeking to clarify the patterns of inheritance and collecting blood samples to isolate the DNA for molecular analysis in search of a "Parkinson" gene. At this time the search is well underway, and there is every reason to believe that the location of such a gene on a particular chromosome may soon be found! Maybe this year, maybe next—but it will be found.

Many patients are aware that a parent, grandparent, aunt or uncle, or perhaps an older brother or sister were also affected with symptoms of Parkinson's disease. Occasionally patients are members of families in which the disease has occurred in several successive generations. We have found that at least one-quarter of our patients know of one or more affected relatives. We have also been able to find among our patients many families with several or more known cases over two or more generations. Many such multiple-case families have been found by other neurologists in the past several years. They are much more common than we had recognized in the past.

Most patients do not know of any affected relatives. They appear to be "sporadic" in contrast to "familial" cases. But there are many reasons why the familial pattern of the disease may escape notice. An important one is the late age of onset. Half of patients have symptom onset after age 75! Thus at least some deceased relatives might have developed symptoms had they lived longer. We often learn that a grandparent who lived a full life and passed on 50 or 60 years ago is remembered to have had a tremor in the last few years of his or her life and perhaps to have walked leaning forward with a shuffling gait, but no one knows whether a diagnosis was ever made. Medical records are not likely to be available. The symptoms may have been ascribed to arthritis, to strokes, or to old age, and the condition may thus have escaped recognition. We may suspect that such a forebear may well have had Parkinson's disease, but of course we cannot be certain.

Many of our patients thought initially to be sporadic have turned out to be familial when more information was discovered on exploring their family trees. In some cases symptoms developed some years later in a parent or a brother or sister. An example is a patient whose mother's parkinsonism appeared in her 80s, 15 years after he began to have symptoms. In other cases an affected family member has concealed the fact. One of our patients, for example, thought he was the only family member to be affected when we first saw him. Ten years later he discovered at a family reunion that a sister he had not seen in many years also had Parkinson's disease. Although they corresponded all those years, she had never told her brother about her Parkinson's. Another patient told me that his brother had tremor of the hands but he never visited him because he didn't want his brother to know of his own affliction.

MULTIPLE-CASE FAMILIES

Only recently have large families with multiple cases of Parkinson's disease been studied in which post-mortem examination of brain tissue has confirmed the diagnosis in at least some affected members. Let's review here several of these families to show how they have shaped our thinking about the genetic aspects of Parkinson's disease and to illustrate the patterns of inheritance that may be found.

The Contursi Kindred

Our associate, Dr. Lawrence Golbe, discovered among our patients an especially large family comprising several hundred persons who shared a common ancestor eleven generations back! That ancestor lived in the 18th century in the small village of Contursi in the Campania, a beautiful mountainous region in Italy south of Mount Vesuvius. Several members of the family migrated to the United States between 1900 and 1920. Some descendants of both the immigrants and those who remained in Italy have Parkinson's disease. Our colleagues at the University of Naples in Italy, Professors Giuseppe Di Iorio and Vincenzo Bonavita studied the Italian branches of the family. Dr. Golbe has studied the American branches. At present a total of 61 persons in several branches of this family are known to have had symptoms of Parkinson's disease in the last 4 generations. About half of these lived all their lives in Italy; the other half lived in the United States, mainly in New York City and adjacent areas. An affected member of this family had consulted one of us (RCD) in 1965 and another in 1980! Still another was a patient of JS. Post-mortem confirmation of the diagnosis was made in two cases. Lewy bodies were present in the appropriate places, leaving no doubt that this is true Parkinson's disease.

The Spellman–Muenter Kindred

Dr. George Spellman, a physician practicing in Sioux City, Iowa, reported in 1962 about a family in which 9 cases of parkinsonism had appeared in 4 generations. Two affected family members had attended the Mayo Clinic in Rochester, Minnesota—one as far back as the 1920s. By family report that patient's grandfather, who died in 1913, had "paralysis agitans." Dr. Manfred Muenter of the Mayo Clinic subsequently encountered additional members of the family. As of 1986, 14 members were known to have been affected in the last 5 generations. By 1993 several additional members were found to have had Parkinson s disease, bringing the total to 22 affected persons. Two family members had only mild tremor, which led Dr. Muenter and Dr. Demetrios Maraganore, his associate, to wonder whether these two had essential tremor! Post-mortem examinations carried out in several affected members of this family leave no doubt that the family disease is true Parkinson's disease.

Other Families

Another similar family was encountered in southern California by Dr. Cheryl Waters, also with post-mortem confirmation of the diagnosis. Three large American families of German and Danish origin were recently described by Dr. Zbigniew Wzollek of the University of Nebraska in Omaha, again with positive post-mortem studies. Dr. Golbe recently studied a family from Pennsylvania in which 7 persons were affected in 4 generations. Post-mortem confirmation of typical Parkinson's disease was obtained in 1 family member.

In an Irish family studied by our colleague Dr. Margery Mark and by Dr. David Brooks at the Hammersmith Hospital in London, positron emission tomography (PET) was used to make the diagnosis in at-risk relatives who had no symptoms. The family consisted of 10 brothers and sisters and their mother. Parkinson symptoms developed in the oldest sibling in his 30s, and he came under the care of RCD. He eventually died of pneumonia. Post-mortem examination of his brain confirmed typical Lewy-body Parkinson's disease. Similar symptoms subsequently developed in his younger brother. Dr. Mark treated him with levodopa/carbidopa, and he responded quite well. She then sent his mother and all the other brothers and sisters, including a sister who lived in London, to Dr. Brooks for PET studies. Dr. Brooks found that the mother and two sisters had impairment of brain dopamine systems in a pattern typical of Parkinson's disease. Thus in addition to the two affected brothers, their mother and two of their sisters also had the disease even though they had no symptoms or physical signs of parkinsonism.

These families, and many others like them, confirm that true Parkinson's disease can occur as a hereditary condition. Further the pattern of inheritance in all these families indicates that a single abnormal gene may be the primary cause. The very existence of these families—and the strikingly similar symptoms in different branches of the same family living in different parts of the world—argue against an environmental factor, whether a virus or a toxin, as a primary cause.

HOW OFTEN IS PARKINSON'S DISEASE FAMILIAL?

To find out how often Parkinson's disease is familial, our clinical geneticist, Alice Lazzarini, questioned all 216 Parkinson's disease patients whom RCD had seen in our clinic during calendar year 1991. She worked with these patients and their families to identify all their first- and second-degree relatives. She called upon all living relatives to find those who might be affected with some Parkinson symptoms. To identify deceased relatives, she obtained birth, marriage, and death certificates in various public registries and tracked down old medical records. We and our colleagues, Dr. Mark, Dr. Golbe, and Dr. Thomas Zimmerman, then examined those living relatives who were reported to have any Parkinson symptoms. We traveled all over the country to visit those unable to come to us.

We found that 26% of the patients had at least one affected relative. The majority had no known affected relatives. They are said to have "sporadic" parkinsonism. However, we also found that most people have little or no information on the fates of their grandparents or all their aunts and uncles. In only 23% could we obtain information on all first- and second-degree relatives, that is, on all brothers and sisters, both parents, all four grandparents, and all aunts and uncles.

It may seem surprising at first that so few patients could give a full account of their families. However, we challenge you, dear reader, to jot down your own family tree and see how well you can do. Chances are, you do not know all your grandparents. Some may have died before you were born or when you were a small child, and you probably have little notion what illnesses they may have had. Most persons have aunts and uncles whose whereabouts have been unknown for many years. Quite a few persons have lost a parent in childhood. Some parents were divorced decades ago, or a father may have abandoned the family when the patient was a child. Some patients have lost large portions of their families in the great wars of the 20th century and in the Holocaust. Finally a small number of patients were orphans.

When our geneticist Lazzarini's analysis considered only those patients who did know about both parents, all brothers and sisters, all four grandparents, and all aunts and uncles, the proportion who had one or more affected relatives rose to about 50%! The true proportion of Parkinson patients whose disease is familial must be even greater than that! Because of the late age at which Parkinson symptoms may first appear, it is likely that some of the relatives who died in their 60s or 70s would have shown signs and symptoms of the disease had they lived longer. In a population survey for Parkinson's disease carried out in the early 1980s, Dr. William Mutch and his colleagues in Glasgow, Scotland, found that the *median* age of onset was in the mid-70s. That means that half of patients had disease onset after age 75. Some patients have their initial symptoms in their 80s; a few in their 90s. We know of one patient whose symptoms first appeared at age 101!

FORMES FRUSTE

We have found in our studies of families that some relatives have very mild symptoms for many years. They have an incompletely developed parkinsonism. Physicians call such cases "formes fruste" (from the French, meaning a condition whose development has been "frustrated"). These persons, with only one or two mild symptoms, had not sought medical attention. If they had, they were not diagnosed as having Parkinson's disease. Some with only tremor as a symptom may be diagnosed with essential tremor. An example is the brother of a patient who had the onset of tremor in his right hand at age 25. When seen at age 82, he still had only tremor of the right hand. A physician himself, he believed that he had essential tremor. But on examination he had a number of telltale signs of Parkinson's disease such as mild rigidity of the muscles of the right arm and loss of the normal swing of that arm on walking. His tremor was also present at rest with a typical pill-rolling character. There can be little question that his correct diagnosis was Parkinson's disease.

A FAMILY DISEASE

As we come to terms with the fact that heredity plays a large role in Parkinson's disease, the patient is no longer the sole subject of attention. The entire family becomes involved. A host of new questions arise. What are the chances that other members may become affected? When? Does the disease skip generations? Can anything be done to identify those at risk? If so, can the disease be prevented?

Unfortunately we can only answer these questions in a general way. We lack as yet the information or the methods to predict which other family members are likely to show Parkinson symptoms later in life. We do not yet have a practical means of diagnosing the disease before symptoms develop. Nor do we presently have the means of preventing the disease from developing. We can only make a rough estimate of the risk of Parkinson symptoms developing in offspring of affected individuals at some time within a normal life span. Some years ago Dr. Leonard Kurland, a neurologist and epidemiologist at the Mayo Clinic, estimated the lifetime risk of Parkinson's disease developing in any individual to be 2.5%. Clearly the risk to offspring of an affected individual will be somewhat greater than that.

The patterns of inheritance found in studying the multi-case families described above show us that Parkinson's disease is, in genetic terms, an *autosomal-dominant* disorder. To explain what this means, it is necessary to briefly review some elements of genetics. Human beings contain 23 pairs of chromosomes in the nucleus of every cell. They were called chromosomes (from the Greek, meaning colored bodies) because they take the color of certain chemical stains that render them visible under the microscope. They exist in pairs, one received from each parent. Two of the chromosomes, named "X" and "Y," are the sex chromosomes.

The remaining 22 pairs of chromosomes are called *autosomes*. Males have a Y chromosome inherited from their fathers and an X inherited from their mothers. Females have two X chromosomes. We can infer that the gene for Parkinson's disease cannot be on either of the sex chromosomes since the disease occurs equally in men and women. Hence it is an "autosomal" disorder.

The term "dominant" indicates that a single copy of the disease gene is sufficient to cause the disease. In contrast there are also "recessive" disorders, such as cystic fibrosis. In autosomal-recessive disorders symptoms of the disorder do *not* develop in individuals carrying a single copy of the disease gene inherited from one parent plus a normal copy inherited from the other parent. These individuals are carriers because they can transmit the gene to their progeny. Symptoms of recessive disorders develop only in those who receive two copies of the disease gene, one copy from each parent. That means both parents must be carriers. In general, as might be expected from this fact, recessive disorders are relatively rare, whereas dominant disorders are more common.

Several researchers, including our colleague Alice Lazzarini and Dr. Maraganore of the Mayo Clinic, have found that affected relatives were nearly always concentrated on one side of a patient's family. For example, if 3 or 4 affected relatives were identified, they were nearly always all on the maternal side or the paternal side. Rarely were they found on both sides of the family. This is in itself a powerful argument in favor of a genetic cause for Parkinson's disease. However, because the disease is not uncommon, one would expect rare cases in which there were affected relatives on both sides of the families. We have seen a small number of patients who had affected relatives on both sides. It seems possible that such individuals might have inherited two copies of the Parkinson gene, one from each parent. Their disease did not seem different from that in other patients. However, we know that in other dominantly inherited conditions, having two copies of the disease gene does not seem to make any difference.

Although each offspring of a parent afflicted with a dominant disorder has a 50% chance of carrying the disease gene, it does not mean that the disease will actually develop in 1 of every 2 offspring. This is because "penetrance" is incomplete. Due to the late age of onset of Parkinson's disease, only some of those who inherit the disease gene are likely to experience symptoms within a normal lifetime. Since we have observed Parkinson's disease first developing at age 101, we can conclude that penetrance will remain incomplete even at age 100!

The risk of Parkinson symptoms developing in a relative of someone with the disease is somewhat more than the 2.5% risk faced by the population as a whole—but it is less than 50%. From the observation that half of patients have disease onset after age 75, we can conclude that the risk of symptoms developing in offspring cannot be more than 25%. From the observation in post-mortem studies of "incidental" Lewy-body disease, we know that there are more subclinical than symptomatic cases (see Chapter 13). Thus the risk must be substantially less than 25%. We would estimate that the actual risk is somewhere between 10 and 15%. We further know that some offspring will experience mild, forme fruste symptoms, which may not justify the clinical diagnosis of Parkinson's disease as now understood.

Taking all these facts and observations into account, we can conclude that— considering all the other diseases and accidents that can happen over the course of a lifetime—the risk of passing Parkinson's disease on to offspring should not be a cause of undue concern. At this time we would not recommend that unaffected relatives or offspring of a patient seek examination in the hope of finding out whether they are affected. Our opinion on this would doubtless be different if we had a reliable and accurate diagnostic test and the means of preventing or delaying the appearance and progression of parkinsonism.

Our new knowledge of the genetics of Parkinson's disease brings hope, but there is still much work to be done.

15

Future Prospects

The introduction of levodopa treatment in the late 1960s resulted from important scientific advances that led to the discovery of dopamine in the brain and its deficiency in parkinsonism. That led logically to the use of levodopa to correct the deficiency, and it worked unexpectedly well. The treatment of Parkinson's disease became rational and far more effective than ever before. There have been many minor refinements and improvements in treatment since then. But all these improvements were based on dopamine deficiency. These included better means of delivering dopamine to the deprived brain regions, as well as drugs imitating the actions of dopamine, or extending or enhancing its actions.

It seems clear that another major advance in treatment can only come from another major advance in our understanding of the fundamental nature of Parkinson's disease. That is, the next major advance in treatment will come from an understanding of the basic mechanisms of the disease process itself. To put it more bluntly, to find a cure we must find the cause. We must find out why those dopamine nerve cells are sick in the first place, so that we can then rationally develop means of correcting or preventing their illness. And we will also need to consider all the other nerve cell systems that are affected in the disease.

That will require a very major advance indeed in our understanding of the disease. It will come from a previously unexpected quarter and from a scientific technology that was developed only in the past decade. That is, it will come from modern molecular genetics.

GENETICS

We now have both the opportunity and the means of reaching the goal that has so long eluded us. The large multiple-case Parkinson families (see Chapter 14) provide us the opportunity. The techniques of modern molecular analysis of DNA provides us the means. Given these families, it is a virtual certainty that the location of the responsible DNA mutation will be found. Indeed scientists in many laboratories throughout the world are already searching for a "Parkinson" gene. The search has already moved through several phases.

At first scientists examined known genes suggested for one theoretical reason or another as the possible site of a variation or mutation that might be linked to Parkinson's disease. As far back as 1971, Dr. William Martin, then at the University of Minnesota, suggested that an inherited defect in the enzyme tyrosine hydroxylase might underlie the dopamine deficiency of parkinsonism (see the discussion of tyrosine in Chapter 7). It is this enzyme that converts tyrosine to L-dopa. If one thought of Parkinson's disease merely as a deficiency of dopamine, then clearly a defect in this enzyme might plausibly be thought to underlie the disease. This line of thought led Dr. H. Tanaka and others at Nigata University, Nigata, Japan (who had isolated the gene that codes for this enzyme) to see whether perhaps there was a defect in that gene in Parkinson patients. They examined the gene for tyrosine hydroxylase in families with multiple cases of parkinsonism. They found no connection and felt they had excluded that possibility.

Dr. Victor McKusick of the Johns Hopkins University School of Medicine suggested in his atlas of human genetic disorders that the cause of Parkinson's disease might be a defect in a gene coding for a system of enzymes in the liver that metabolize drugs and toxins. The gene for one of these enzymes, called debrisoquin hydroxylase, is now known. Large series of patients were studied to see if one of the many known variants of this gene was consistently associated with Parkinson's disease. This was an intriguing idea and a relatively simple one to study, but no definite association has been found.

The theory that an MPTP-like substance (see discussion of MPTP in Chapter 13) might be involved has led other geneticists to examine the genes for monoamine oxidase, the enzyme that converts MPTP to its toxic analog MPP^+. The results so far from half a dozen research groups have failed to find a definite link.

Dr. Thomas Gasser of the University of Munich, Germany, Dr. William Johnson, director of the William Dow Lovett Laboratory of Molecular Neurogenetics at Robert Wood Johnson Medical School in New Jersey, and many other geneticists working in laboratories throughout the world have been testing these various "candidate" genes. So far none has been found guilty of the dubious distinction of being the Parkinson gene.

In this initial phase geneticists have studied a number of known genes suggested by theories about the disease. Their negative findings have essentially excluded all these "candidate" genes and the related hypotheses. Now geneticists are advancing to the next phase. Recognizing that we have no clues to the possible location of the Parkinson gene, they are systematically searching the entire human genome. Many mutations responsible for human disease have been found in this way in the past decade. It is a tedious task, but with modern methods of DNA analysis it can be done. It is only a matter of time before these researchers find the location of the gene defect responsible for Parkinson's disease. They may find it this year or maybe next, but they will surely find it! And then, in the language of baseball, "it will be a whole new ball game."

The discovery of the site of a DNA mutation on a region of a particular chromosome will be the beginning of a new era. Then we will have a marker for the disease that could be used for diagnosis. A reliable DNA marker will enable us to confirm the diagnosis in early and doubtful cases, for example in patients who only have tremor of the hands. Initially the test will be used in all patients who might conceivably have Parkinson's disease. Indeed a reliable DNA marker will make it possible to diagnose Parkinson's disease in the absence of parkinsonism or even in the absence of any signs or symptoms at all. That is, presymptomatic diagnosis will be possible.

While a reliable diagnostic blood test will undoubtedly be an important advance in itself, it may prove to be a Pandora's box, full of problems as well as of opportunities. Without the medical capability of stopping or even slowing the disease process, presymptomatic diagnosis may not always be desirable. Few would really want to know whether or not they have the Parkinson gene and are thus at risk of developing parkinsonism at some unknown time in the future if there is little that can be done to prevent it. We will need to consider under what conditions the test should be used. Appropriate guidelines will need to be developed. Genetic counseling will become part of the medical management of Parkinson's disease.

Fortunately the story will not end here. The real reason for chasing the Parkinson gene is to ultimately find a means of cure and prevention. The discovery of DNA markers closely linked to the disease will be quickly followed by further research to identify the specific piece of DNA affected and which changes in the DNA code cause the disease and which changes prevent it. Very probably the mutation will prove to be in the DNA sequence for a particular gene; perhaps it will be a gene that is already known but more probably one still unknown. The specific protein encoded by the gene will be synthesized. Very probably it will be a protein that is presently unknown. Perhaps it will be named "parkinsin." Scientists will try to determine what that protein normally does, how the defect alters its structure and function, and how it causes disease. This knowledge will lead to new forms of treatment undreamable today.

We can only speculate at present as to how a gene defect might cause Parkinson's disease. Some geneticists believe that the disease is "multifactorial"; that is, both genetic and environmental factors must interact to produce the disease. They believe that what is inherited is a predisposition to the disease's developing in certain circumstances. Others argue that diseases such as Parkinson's disease, Alzheimer's disease, and others of adult onset are "polygenic"; that is, they reflect the action of several genes. For example, there could be a principal disease gene, but other genes may facilitate or inhibit its expression. Another view is that a single gene will be found responsible for most cases and that differences between patients will be explained by differences in the size of the defect in that particular gene.

NERVE GROWTH FACTORS

Proteins somewhat like insulin have been found to play an important role in regulating the growth of nerve cells and in maintaining them throughout life. These have been called "nerve growth factors" (NGF), or neurotrophins. One of these factors, called "sympathetic nerve growth factor," was first discovered a half century ago by Dr. Rita Levi–Montalcini of Italy. This substance was at first thought to act only on the sympathetic nerves. Later, however, it was found to stimulate the growth of the cholinergic nerve cells in the brain, specifically those in a cluster of cells in the upper brainstem called the *nucleus basalis of Meynert*. The cells of this nucleus are affected in Alzheimer's disease, and their loss is thought to underlie the memory impairments typical of that condition. These cells are also affected in Parkinson's disease. More recently other NGFs that act on the dopamine nerve cells of the substantia nigra have been found. Among these are "brain-derived" NGF (BDNGF) and "glial-derived" NGF (GDNGF). Both of these received much attention at first, and it was suggested they might be used to treat Parkinson's disease.

Direct administration of NGFs has been attempted experimentally in animal models and in patients with a variety of nervous system disorders. Administration of NGF directly into the brain has been attempted experimentally in the treatment of Alzheimer's disease, but the results are not satisfactory. Another factor called "ciliary growth factor" has been tried in amyotrophic lateral sclerosis (Lou Gehrig's disease)—again without definite benefit. In fact it appeared to make some cases worse. An NGF has also been tried in diabetics with peripheral nerve involvement. There has been some discussion of the possibility of testing BDNGF and GDNGF in Parkinson patients, but so far no trial has been planned.

Because these factors are proteins, they can reach their target nerve cells only if injected directly into the brain. They do not spread through the brain, so they must be injected very near the target nerve cells. Thus researchers are turning to indirect methods of inducing the brain to produce more such factors. Unfortunately the nerve growth factors have turned out to be far more complicated than had initially been suspected. There are entire families and subfamilies of these factors. Each type of nerve cell and each nucleus of brain cells appear to have its own specific family of such factors, yet these factors act at many different sites. In view of the multiplicity of NGFs and the complexity of their actions neuroscientists will need to learn a great deal more about them. We can only speculate at this time whether manipulation of NGFs may lead to new therapeutic approaches to Parkinson's disease. There is at present no evidence of a deficiency of an NGF in Parkinson patients.

THE MEANING OF THE LEWY BODY

Thinking on the cause of Parkinson's disease is beginning to take into account the relatively large number of "pre-diagnosable" cases and the widespread distribution of Lewy bodies in the nervous system. It appears that Lewy-body disease can produce different sets of symptoms. Most of the time it produces no symptoms at all, but when it does, it usually produces the symptoms that we know as "Parkinson's disease." Yet sometimes it produces a condition indistinguishable from Alzheimer's disease with or without parkinsonian symptoms, and not infrequently it produces a Parkinson-like condition with unusual features. Thus when we have found the cause of Lewy-body disease, we will have found the cause of Parkinson's disease.

It seems likely that the Lewy body is the result of the disease process rather than its cause. Nevertheless, if we understood how and why the neurofilaments of the diseased nerve cells formed these abnormal bundles, we would have made valuable progress toward understanding the mechanism of the disease process. Unfortunately it is very difficult to study the formation of these bundles. As yet no means of inducing them in experimental animals has been found. Despite the difficulties research on the fundamental structure and chemical composition of the Lewy body is gradually increasing.

Recently it has been found that Lewy bodies contain a protein named "ubiquitin." Using antibodies to ubiquitin to help them see Lewy bodies under the microscope, neuropathologists are now finding that these bodies are more numerous and widespread in the brain than had previously been realized. This new tool will greatly stimulate research directed at defining the range of disorders in which Lewy bodies may be found. We can expect profound changes in our concepts of the various conditions associated with Lewy bodies.

NEW DRUGS

Although over two dozen dopamine receptor agonists have been tried in parkinsonism thus far and all appear to be about equivalent, it is possible that better agonists may yet be found. The gene coding for the dopamine receptor has been identified; it is located on chromosome 11. It can now be cloned in the laboratory, and the intimate structure of the receptor protein can be studied in far greater detail than was previously possible. This will facilitate the search for new drugs designed to activate the receptor and could consequently lead to a new generation of dopamine receptor agonists.

TRANSPLANTATION

While experimental brain transplants will continue and improvements in technique will lead to better results, transplant surgery will remain experimental for the foreseeable future, certainly beyond the turn of the century. The development of genetically engineered cell lines will obviate the need for fetal cells. The pursuit of transplant therapy will lead in other, as yet unexpected directions. For example, it may become possible to take some of the patients' own cells and, by gene-splicing techniques, transfer to them the capacity to make L-dopa or perhaps even dopamine and then return them to the patient. The identification of a gene defect in Parkinson's disease will put the question of transplantation in a new perspective. Researchers will focus on transplantation of the missing gene or portion thereof by some means—with the prospect of correcting all defects of the disease, not merely the deficiency in dopamine-producing cells.

Appendix 1

Drug Finder

The most commonly prescribed anti-Parkinson drugs are listed in Tables 1 and 2, with a brief description of dosages and formulations.

Most tablets and capsules have distinctive shapes, markings, coloring, and code numbers to facilitate identification. The letters and numbers are often very small, and a magnifying glass may be needed to read them. Some manufacturers impress the company name on their tablets and capsules. The Du Pont name appears on the red Symmetrel (amantadine) capsule, and the Roche name on the Madopar (benserazide/levodopa) capsule. Others manufacturers print an initial or an identifying trademark or logo on their products. Lederle Laboratories, for example, has an L in script on the front of each tablet. Merck, Sharp & Dohme products

TABLE 1. *Commonly prescribed anti-Parkinson drugs*

Brand (trade) name	Generic name	Formulations
Anticholinergics		
Akineton	Biperiden	2 mg white tablet
Artane	Trihexyphenidyl	2 and 5 mg white tablets and 5 mg long-acting capsules
Cogentin	Benztropine	0.5 and 2 mg round white tablets and 1 mg long elliptical white tablets
Kemadrin	Procyclidine	2 and 5 mg white tablets
Symmetrel	Amantadine	100 mg bright red capsule
Dopamine receptor agonists		
Dopergine[a]	Lisuride	0.2 mg, 0.5 mg, 1 mg white scored tablets
Parlodel	Bromocriptine	2.5 mg tablets and 5 mg capsules, caramel and white
Permax	Pergolide	0.05 mg ivory; 0.25 mg green, and 1 mg pink tablets; rectangular scored
Type B monoamine oxidase inhibitors		
Eldepryl	Selegiline (deprenyl)	5 mg white round scored tablets

[a] Not available in the United States.

TABLE 2. *Levodopa preparations available in the United States and Canada*

Brand (trade) name	Generic name	Formulations
Levodopa alone Larodopa	Levodopa	Pink tablets[a] 0.1 gram (elliptical, scored) 0.25 gram (round) 0.5 gram (oblong, scored) Capsules 0.1 gram (pink and scarlet) 0.25 gram (pink and beige) 0.5 gram (pink)
Levodopa–decarboxylase inhibitor combinations Madopar	Benserazide/levodopa	Capsules 25/100 mg (pink and blue) 50/200 mg (caramel and blue) Dispersible tablets "625" 12.5/50 mg (pink tablets) "125" 25/100 mg (pink tablets)
Madopar HBS[b] 125	Benserazide/levodopa	Capsules 25/100 mg (blue and black)
Sinemet	Carbidopa/levodopa	Elliptical tablets, scored 10/100 mg (dark dapple blue) 25/250 mg (light dapple blue) 25/100 mg (yellow)
Sinemet CR[b]	Carbidopa/levodopa	50/200 mg (peach) 25/100 mg (pink, not scored)

[a] Note: 0.1 gram = 100 mg; 0.25 gram = 250 mg; and 0.5 gram = 500 mg.
[b] These preparations of Madopar and Sinemet are sustained-release (also called controlled-release or slow-release) formulations.

have the letters MSD in boldface above an identifying three-digit number, and Sandoz marks an S within a triangle. Tablets are usually scored on the reverse side so that they can easily be broken in half for smaller doses. The pattern of the scoring is often distinctive.

Despite all these distinguishing features, some pills may be difficult to identify. If there is any doubt about the identity of a forgotten bottle of pills, discard it or consult a pharmacist before using the drug.

Appendix 2

Organizations Concerned with Parkinson's Disease

NATIONAL INSTITUTES OF HEALTH

The National Institute of Neurological Disorders and Stroke (NINDS) in Bethesda, Maryland, plays an important role in Parkinson's disease. NINDS is one of the National Institutes of Health (NIH), the major United States government agency engaged in medical research and a part of the Department of Health and Human Services. The director of the NIH reports directly to the Surgeon General of the U.S. Public Health Service.

NINDS and other NIH institutes maintain a program of research in their own research laboratories and an active program of clinical research at the Clinical Center, a large hospital and clinic also located in Bethesda. A small number of patients are accepted there for special investigations and trials of new forms of treatment, including experimental drugs. Most important, NIH has trained many scientists who have gone on to become leaders in biomedical research in universities and research institutes throughout the world. It also sponsors a large-scale program of research grants to scientists at universities and research laboratories throughout the country. Some of these grants support research in Parkinson's disease and related conditions and basic research relevant to these disorders. For example, the NIH sponsored the Deprenyl and Tocopherol Antioxidant Therapy of Parkinsonism (DATATOP) study.

As we mentioned in Chapter 13, it was the fundamental biochemical work of Dr. Julius Axelrod and his colleagues at the NINDS in the 1950s that made possible the discovery of dopamine in the brain and its deficiency in Parkinson's disease. Dr. Axelrod won the Nobel Prize in Medicine for his achievements in this field. Most of the scientists who worked on brain dopamine in the 1960s had studied with Dr. Axelrod. After his retirement this work was continued by Dr. Irving Kopin and his colleagues, including Dr. Thomas Chase. In the 1970s the NINDS established the Experimental Therapeutics Branch headed by Dr. Donald Calne, who with these fellows carried out many clinical drug trials and played a major role in the development of treatment with dopamine receptor agonists such as bromocriptine. Subsequently Dr. Chase became Director of the Experimental Therapeutics Branch and carried out extensive studies on the metabolism and mechanism of action of levodopa in parkinsonism. The late Dr. Bruce Schoenberg, who directed the Neuroepidemiology Branch of NINDS, carried out important studies on the prevalence of Parkinson's disease in different regions of the world.

The NINDS makes available an annual summary of research in Parkinson's disease; it is prepared each January. A free informational booklet on Parkinson's disease is also available. Currently this is NIH publication No. 94-139 entitled *Parkinson's Disease, Hope Through Research*. It was last updated September 1994. Copies may be obtained by writing to the Office of Scientific and Health Reports, NINDS, Building 31, Room 8A16, National Institutes of Health, Bethesda MD, 20892. One may call the office at (301) 496-5751.

Unfortunately because of gradual reductions in funding, the role of the NIH in research has gradually diminished. It must be admitted that the NIH now provides limited support to research in Parkinson's disease. Recently NINDS has been funding less than 15% of research grant applications approved for scientific merit. The consequences for biomedical research have been little less than devastating. As a result Parkinson's disease research has become mainly dependent on funding from the private sector, chiefly pharmaceutical firms, the nonprofit voluntary agencies, and private philanthropy.

Voluntary agencies have been active for some years in sponsoring research in Parkinson's disease, providing information and educational materials, newsletters, and educational symposia for patients and their families. In the United States there are several agencies operating at a national level, plus many large regional associations or foundations. There are also hundreds of local organizations, some affiliated with one of the national organizations and others operated by the patient-education divisions of local hospitals or functioning independently.

Repeated efforts have been made over the years to merge these agencies into one single national organization comparable to those operating in other fields such as heart disease, multiple sclerosis, or epilepsy. So far these efforts have met with little success. This fact may explain why governmental sponsorship of research in Parkinson's disease has been much less extensive than that devoted to other diseases of comparable prevalence.

The major North American agencies are the following:

The American Parkinson Disease Association, Inc.
1250 Hylan Boulevard
Staten Island, NY 10305
Tel: (718) 981-8001, (800) 223-2732; fax: (718) 981-4300

West Coast regional office:
The American Parkinson Disease Association, Inc.
15000 Ventura Boulevard, #384
Sherman Oaks, CA 91403
Tel: (818) 906-7108

Washington, DC, regional office:
The American Parkinson Disease Association, Inc.
807 South Alfred Street, #2
Alexandria, VA 22314
Tel: (703) 684-1108

The Parkinson's Disease Foundation
William Black Medical Research Building
650-710 West 168th Street
New York, NY 10032
Tel: (212) 923-4700, (800) 457-6676; fax: (212) 923-4778

The National Parkinson Foundation, Inc.
1501 Ninth Avenue/Bob Hope Road
Miami, FL 33136
Tel: (305) 547-6666; Information lines: (800) 327-4545; in Florida: (800) 433-7022; in California: (800) 400-8448

United Parkinson Foundation
833 West Washington Boulevard
Chicago, IL 60607
Tel: (312) 733-1893

The Parkinson Foundation of Canada
Suite 232 ManuLife Centre
55 Bloor Street West
Toronto, Ontario, Canada M4W 1A6

The **American Parkinson Disease Association (APDA)**, founded in the early 1960s, grew rapidly to a national organization with chapters in many cities. Presently, Salvatore Esposite serves as president. Paul Maestrone, DVM, is the scientific director. Roger C. Duvoisin, M.D., has recently been appointed chairman of the Scientific Advisory Board. The board comprises leading scientists in various biomedical fields. The APDA maintains a booth at the annual meetings of the American Academy of Neurology.

The APDA supports a national program of clinics and information centers throughout the United States. The information centers provide support and liaison to local support groups located in their areas. With the help of the national office, the local chapters organize patient education symposia featuring presentations by leading researchers in the field of Parkinson's disease. The association also publishes a quarterly newsletter, booklets, and other informational materials. One booklet describes a program of exercises for use at home and another outlining various aids and adaptive equipment for home use.

In addition to patient service, the association also sponsors a program of research at institutions throughout the country. Its Scientific Advisory Board meets annually to review research grant applications submitted to the Association. From among the many submitted, the advisory board selects the most promising for funding. These include 1-year grants and 3-year "century grants." In addition the APDA sponsors the prestigious George Cotzias Fellowship, which provides both research support and a stipend to promising young scientists for 3 years. Typically the Cotzias Fellows are young neurologists who have completed their clinical training plus a period of research training and are ready to begin their own research under the supervision of a scientist in a major university or research institute. A number of prominent investigators, for example, Dr. G. Frederick Wooten, Professor and Chairman of Neurology at the University of Virginia Medical School, began their careers as Cotzias Fellows. The APDA also supports advanced research centers at leading institutions providing core support to groups of scientists working on Parkinson's disease. Our own Parkinson research group was designated an APDA Advanced Research Center in 1991. It was the second center to be so designated. At present 8 such centers have been established in the United States.

The **Parkinson's Disease Foundation** was established in 1957 by the late William Black for the purpose of supporting scientific research into the cause of Parkinson's disease with the hope of eventually finding a cure or a means of prevention. Mr. Black also provided a gift to Columbia University, which funded the construction of a research tower, the William Black Medical Research Building, one floor of which was dedicated to research on Parkinson's disease and houses the Foundation's offices and core research laboratories. An active research program is based in these laboratories. Over the years the Foundation has played an important role in advancing research in Parkinson's disease. In its first years it quietly funded basic research on the chemistry and metabolism of L-dopa and later funded one of the initial clinical trials of levodopa carried out at the Columbia–Presbyterian Medical Center in New York. It helped fund the first American twin study led by RCD.

Dr. Stanley Fahn, a world-renowned authority on Parkinson's disease, serves as scientific director. Dr. Lewis P. Rowland, the distinguished Lucy Moses Professor and Chairman of the Department of Neurology at the College of Physicians and Surgeons of Columbia University, is the Foundation's president. A panel of distinguished leaders in the field served on the Research Advisory Board. Under the direction of its able executive director, Mrs. Dinah Tottenham Orr, the Foundation publishes a newsletter and sponsors periodic symposia for physicians and caregivers. Mrs. Orr also often represents the Foundation at major scientific meetings dealing with Parkinson's disease.

The **National Parkinson Foundation (NPF)** was established in 1957 by the late S. Jay Levey in Miami, Florida. It has long been ably directed by its chairman, Mr. Nathan Slewett. Its officers include Mr. Emilio Alonso-Mednoza, national director, and Harold Kravitz, Esq., president. Over the years the NPF has enjoyed the support of show business celebrities, including Bob Hope (honorary national chairman), Dick Clark, and Phyllis Diller, in its fund-raising activities.

Initially, the NPF devoted its energies primarily to operating an outpatient treatment and research facility in Miami, which is presently directed by Dr. William

Wiener and affiliated with the Department of Neurology of the University of Miami School of Medicine. Subsequently it began to provide research grants to investigators throughout the United States and has established a Scientific Advisory Board consisting of leading scientists in the field. Ten years ago it began to identify and support centers of excellence and currently the NPF supports research at 25 centers in the United States plus one at Juntendo University Medical School in Tokyo. The Foundation has sponsored a number of international symposia on the treatment of Parkinson's disease and published the resulting proceedings. It publishes a quarterly newsletter for patients and their families and useful informational pamphlets.

The **United Parkinson Foundation (UPF)** was founded in Chicago in 1963 by Edgar N. Greenebaum, Jr., to provide patients and their families with the knowledge needed to understand Parkinson's disease. It is funded by contributions from the general public, including membership dues. Its medical director, Harold Klawans, MD, is an internationally recognized authority on Parkinson's disease and was for many years the director of the Parkinson's Disease Research Center at Rush–Presbyterian–St. Luke's Medical Center in Chicago.

Judy Rosner, its executive director, and her assistant, Ms. Jeanne Lee, regularly attend both national and international neurological meetings and maintain personal contacts with leading scientists throughout the world. They may be found each year at the UPF booth at the annual meetings of the American Academy of Neurology.

A major portion of the UPF's operating expenses is allocated to patient services. These include literature, exercise materials, and a quarterly newsletter mailed to all members. Two half-hour videotapes and the UPF exercise program with accompanying audio tapes are also available. Beginning with a series of symposia in Chicago, the Foundation has sponsored many patient-education meetings throughout the country. Questions and requests for literature may be sent to the Foundation's Chicago office. Patients may write to obtain a personal response to specific problems or referrals to clinical neurologists with a known interest and expertise in Parkinson's disease.

Monies raised over operating costs are used to fund grants to support research in Parkinson's disease. Grant applications are reviewed by a Scientific Advisory Board consisting of leading scientists in the field. Support has been provided for research projects at many clinics and universities throughout the world. The Foundation established a professorial chair in Parkinson's disease at Rush–Presbyterian–St. Luke's Medical Center in Chicago.

Recently the UPF has helped start a foundation for patients with essential tremor. The International Tremor Foundation (ITF) is headed by Dr. William Koller, Professor and Chairman of Neurology at the University of Kansas. Inquiries to the ITF may be directed to the UPF offices in Chicago.

The **Parkinson Foundation of Canada** was founded in the 1960s to provide service to patients and raise funds to support research. In 1979 it established a Parkinson Professorship at the Playfair Neurosciences Unit of the University of Toronto at the Toronto Western Hospital. A network of local chapters and self-help groups has been developed to provide therapy, educational meetings, and discussion sessions to help patients and their families cope with the disease. Educational materials including books, tapes, and informational pamphlets are made available to members and the public. The Foundation also publishes a regular bulletin. It makes a substantial number of research grants to scientists working on Parkinson's disease throughout Canada.

Voluntary agencies have also developed in Japan, the United Kingdom, Italy, Germany, South Africa, and in many other countries. There is not enough space here to list all these organizations. Many are members of the International Federation of Parkinson Societies.

Parkinson patients in Great Britain can obtain help and information from the **Parkinson's Disease Society of the United Kingdom,** 36 Portland Place, London W1N 3DG, UK (tel: 071-255-2432). The society was formed in 1969 by patients, relatives, and friends led by the late "Mali" Jenkins. Their goal was to help patients and their relatives cope with the problems arising from the Parkinson's disease, to collect and disseminate information, and to encourage and provide funds for research. The Society has prospered and grown to a nationwide organization of over 200 branches throughout the UK. Presently it is ably led by its executive director, Mrs. Mary Baker. Like her American counterparts, she also attends international scientific meetings concerned with Parkinson's disease. We recently met her, for example, at the third International Congress of Movement Disorders, in Orlando, Florida.

Early on the Society published a useful monograph written in laymen's language entitled "Parkinson's Disease—A Booklet for Patients and Their Families." Presently it issues a newsletter several times a year. It also raises funds to support research. A major contribution has been a "brain bank," maintained in London. This has made possible important advances in our understanding of the brain pathology of Parkinson's disease, notably the Lewy body. The Society periodically sponsors scientific conferences that bring together researchers from throughout the world to report on recent advances in knowledge and treatment of the disease.

PATIENT SUPPORT GROUPS

Many regional and local foundations have been formed by patients and their families with the view of exchanging ideas and sharing advice on means of coping with practical problems. Some of these self-help or support groups have attained substantial size and prominence in their areas. Examples include the Dallas Area Parkinson Society, the Parkinson Association of the Rockies in Denver, Colorado, the California Parkinson Foundation, and the Parkinson Society of Greater Washington (PSGW) in Washington, DC.

The late Dr. Sidney Dorros, author of an excellent autobiographical account of his experience with parkinsonism, was one of the prime movers of the Parkinson Society of Greater Washington (PSGW). In 1981 the PSGW hosted a national convention of Parkinson support groups at which a national organization was initiated—The Parkinson Support Groups of America (PSGA). This organization was primarily interested in self-help and in developing grassroots support for the formation of a Congressional committee on Parkinson's disease. Although several resolutions to that effect were introduced in Congress, none has passed. The PSGA survives today in a number of local chapters, notably one in Montclair, New Jersey.

There are countless small local support groups in various stages of development. No less than 17 are presently functioning in the state of New Jersey alone! They generally publish newsletters for their members, hold regular meetings, provide exercise sessions, and invite physicians, psychologists, nutritionists, and others to lecture on recent development relevant to parkinsonism. In this way they provide valuable assistance to many patients and their families. The patient-education departments of community hospitals often provide some assistance and space for these local groups. Our own hospital sponsors several groups including one for caregivers and another for young parkinsonians. Some groups also raise funds to support research programs at various medical schools. They thus provide their members an opportunity to participate directly in the ultimate conquest of Parkinson's disease.

THE SOCIETY FOR PROGRESSIVE SUPRANUCLEAR PALSY

A small proportion of patients with parkinsonism in fact suffer from a distinct disorder known as progressive supranuclear palsy (PSP) or Steele–Richardson–Olszewski syndrome. Generally patients with this disorder have participated in the activities of the various Parkinson's disease agencies. However, the Society for Progressive Supranuclear Palsy, Inc., was founded in 1989 by David Saks to focus specifically on the needs of PSP patients, family members, and caregivers. The Society is dedicated to stimulating research in PSP and informing members of recent findings. It publishes a quarterly newsletter, the "PSP Advocate," for patients and their families and makes available several information folders. A booklet "Progressive Supranuclear Palsy: Some Answers" by Dr. Lawrence Golbe is available in English and Spanish. Videotapes in VHS format are also available.

The Society has recently cosponsored several international scientific conferences dealing with PSP, including a diagnostic workshop (held at the NIH) directed by Dr. Irene Litvan. Its executive office is presently at Johns Hopkins Hospital, 5065 Outpatient Center, 601 North Caroline Street, Baltimore, MD 21287.

THE PARKINSON'S WEB

The Parkinson's web is an international, nonprofit effort to use the Internet as an on-line archive of Parkinson's disease information written specifically for patients, their families, friends and caregivers. In addition to general information, this archive will provide information about Parkinson's disease, its treatment, strategies for coping, and research news.

The project is supported by Dr. Anne Young, the Chief of Neurology at the Massachusetts General Hospital, Dr. Jack Penny, and Mr. John Lester. World Wide Web (WWW) users should use the following Universal Resource Locator (URL) to see currently available information: **http://demOnmac.mgh.harvard.edu/ parkinsonsweb/Main/PDmain.html.**

For further information contact Ken Bernstein, president of the Young Parkinson's Chapter of Massachusetts and coordinator of the Parkinson's Web: tel: (617) 527-2803; fax: (617) 527-2077; or e-mail: cocosolo@aol.com.

Glossary

Acetylcholine: Chemical messenger released by the cholinergic nerves, such as the vagus nerve.

Adrenaline (also known as **epinephrine**): Hormone secreted by the adrenal gland into the circulation in moments of crisis. It stimulates the heart to beat faster and work harder, increases the flow of blood to the muscles, causes an increased alertness of mind, and produces other changes to prepare the body to meet an emergency.

Alpha-tocopherol: Chemical name for vitamin E.

Angina pectoris: A characteristic pain in the chest felt as a squeezing or pressing behind the breastbone. It arises in the heart muscle usually during some activity and subsides with rest. It is a symptom of coronary arteriosclerosis or arteriosclerotic heart disease. The pain occurs when the heart muscle, as a result of impaired blood flow in the coronary arteries, fails to receive sufficient oxygen to carry on the work it is called on to do. Pains in muscles of the shoulder and chest are sometimes confused with angina pectoris.

Anticholinergic: Adjective applied to drugs opposing the action of acetylcholine.

Antihistamine: Term applied to drugs opposing the actions of histamine and commonly used to treat allergic disorders such as hay fever and bronchial asthma.

Athetosis: Form of dyskinesia (see below) characterized by involuntary writhing movements usually of the hands or feet. The movements are similar to but slower than those of chorea (see below).

Benign essential tremor: Condition characterized by tremor of the hands, head, voice, and sometimes other parts of the body. It often runs in families and is sometimes called *familial tremor* and *senile tremor* in the elderly. It is sometimes mistaken for Parkinson's disease although there is no rigidity or bradykinesia (see below).

Bradykinesia: Descriptive term meaning slowness of movement (from the Greek *brady*, meaning slow; and *kinesis*, meaning movement); it is a cardinal sign of Parkinson's disease.

Choline: A naturally occurring substance that is a precursor of acetylcholine.

Chorea: Diagnostic term (from the Greek *choreia*, meaning dance) applied to a nervous affection marked by excessive motor activity ranging in severity from restlessness, fidgetiness, and twitching to flinging movements, sudden jerks,

169

and spasms; it is sometimes associated with mental agitation. It is popularly
known as St. Vitus' dance.

Corpus striatum: Anatomical term (from the Latin, meaning striate body) designating a large mass of gray matter deep in each cerebral hemisphere. Its internal structure and function are not yet well understood, but it is believed essentially to modulate or regulate motor and sensory activities of the brain.

Decarboxylase inhibitors: Drugs that inhibit or prevent the action of the enzyme
dopa decarboxylase and thus hinder the conversion of dopa to dopamine. Carbidopa and benserazide (used individually in combination with levodopa) are
decarboxylase inhibitors.

Dopa: Chemical short name for 3,4-dihydroxyphenylalanine, an amino acid occurring in animals and plants. It exists in two forms, the L- and the D-forms (L
being short for the Latin *laevo*, meaning left; and D being short for *dextro*,
meaning right). Only the L-form occurs in nature (see Levodopa).

Dopa decarboxylase: Enzyme found in the nervous system and blood vessels
that controls the metabolic conversion of dopa to dopamine.

Dopamine: Substance derived from dopa in certain nerve cells. It works in the
nervous system as a chemical messenger transmitting impulses from one nerve
cell to the next; it is deficient in Parkinson's disease.

Dyskinesia: General term meaning an abnormal involuntary movement.

Dystonia: Type of involuntary movement that is slow and twisting, and is associated with forceful muscle contractions or spasms. The painful end-of-dose
foot cramp is a common example.

Encephalitis: Inflammation of the brain (from the Greek *encephalon,* meaning
brain; and the suffix *-itis*, meaning inflammation, as in tonsillitis, appendicitis,
etc.); it is usually caused by a virus infection.

Encephalitis lethargica: Type of encephalitis that occurred in scattered epidemics throughout the world from 1916 to 1926. It usually caused sleepiness,
double vision, trouble swallowing, and drooling in the acute phase, and a special type of parkinsonism in its chronic phase. The disorder was also called *von
Economo's encephalitis* (see below) and *epidemic encephalitis.*

Festination: Walking in rapid, short, shuffling steps (from the Latin *festinare*,
meaning to hasten).

Glaucoma: Disorder of the eye characterized by a sustained increase of pressure within the eyeball that can injure the optic nerve and cause impaired
vision.

Globus Pallidum: Anatomical structure of brain, a component of the corpus striatum. It is the target of an operation done to relieve some symptoms of Parkinson's disease.

Lateropulsion: Involuntary stepping or staggering to one side; it occurs in Parkinson's disease but can also be a symptom of inflammation of the inner ear.

Lecithin: Naturally occurring substance containing phosphatidylcholine; it may
be taken by mouth to provide choline to the nervous system to increase the synthesis of the chemical messenger acetylcholine.

Levodopa: International generic name for the medicinal formulation of L-dopa (*laevo* from the Latin, meaning left) (see **Dopa**). It is currently the most effective substance available for the treatment of Parkinson's disease.

Lewy bodies: Round masses (about the size of a red blood cell) surrounded by a clear halo, or vacuole (open space), within affected nerve cells in the substantia nigra and other areas of the brain in patients with Parkinson's disease. They are a microscopic hallmark of the disease, identified in 1908 by Frederic H. Lewy, a German-born neurologist.

Livido reticularis: A purplish or bluish mottling of the skin seen usually around the knee and sometimes on the forearm in patients under treatment with the drug amantadine.

Micrographia: The small handwriting characteristic of many Parkinson's disease patients.

Monoamine oxidase inhibitor (also known as MAO inhibitor): General term applied to a group of drugs that inhibit the enzyme that oxidizes dopamine, adrenaline, and related substances in the body. Drugs in this group enhance the effects of these chemical messengers and have mainly been used in the treatment of depression.

Multiple system atrophy: Medical term used to denote a group of disorders sometimes resembling Parkinson's disease. Various brain systems, though mainly the cerebellum, are affected.

Oculogyria: Spasm of the eye muscles causing the eyes to look upward (rarely downward) involuntarily; it is a characteristic symptom of post-encephalitic parkinsonism following encephalitis lethargica. It has a sudden onset and may last for minutes to hours. Sometimes it occurs as a reaction to certain tranquilizing drugs, but it is never seen in Parkinson's disease.

On–off effect: Descriptive term used to refer to marked, often rapid fluctuations from a state of parkinsonism to a state of normal movement and back again, which may occur several times a day. The effect takes its name from patients' comparing the experience to an electric switch being turned on or off.

Palilalia: Symptom of parkinsonism, especially the post-encephalitic form, in which a word or syllable is repeated several to many times and the flow of speech is interrupted.

Pallidotomy: Operation, done by stereotactic surgery (see below) in which a small region of the Globus Pallidum is destroyed to relieve tremor, rigidity, muscle spasms, and involuntary movements in Parkinson's disease.

Pallidum: See Globus Pallidum.

Paradoxical kinesia: Sudden, usually brief episodes of marked remission of symptoms of parkinsonism that may last minutes, sometimes hours, and rarely several days.

Paralysis agitans: Formerly the official diagnostic term for Parkinson's disease of the World Health Organization's International Statistical Classification of Diseases. It is the Latin form of the older, popular term *shaking palsy* (see below), which was used to describe the disease in James Parkinson's time.

Paresthesia (plural: paresthesias): Sensations, usually unpleasant, arising spontaneously in a limb or other part of the body and variously experienced as "pins and needles" or a feeling of warmth or coldness (thermal paresthesias).

Parkinson's disease: Form of parkinsonism originally described by James Parkinson: a chronic, slowly progressive disease of the nervous system characterized clinically by the combination of tremor, rigidity, bradykinesia, and stooped posture, and pathologically by loss of the pigmented nerve cells of the substantia nigra and the presence of Lewy bodies (see above) within the affected nerve cells.

Parkinsonism: Group of neurological disorders characterized by tremor, rigidity, bradykinesia, stooped posture, and shuffling gait. The more common forms are Parkinson's disease and a reversible syndrome induced by major tranquilizing drugs.

Phenothiazines: Class of drugs extensively employed in medical practice for various purposes. One group includes anti-histaminic agents (e.g., Phenergan) and anti-Parkinson drugs (e.g., ethopropazine). Another larger group comprises the major tranquilizers (e.g., chlorpromazine) that can induce a Parkinson-like state.

Progressive supranuclear palsy: Chronic disorder of the nervous system that often mimics Parkinson's disease. It was first described by Steele, Richardson, and Olszewski in 1964.

Propulsion: Disturbance of gait typical of parkinsonism in which the patient, while walking, steps faster and faster with progressively shorter steps, and then passes from a walking to a running pace and may fall forward.

Retropulsion: Involuntary stepping backward; the reverse of propulsion.

Rigidity (also called **plastic rigidity**): Descriptive term referring to the type of muscular stiffness encountered in Parkinson's disease patients. It is characterized by a constant, even resistance to passive manipulation of the limbs. It is due to a failure of reciprocal relaxation of the antagonist muscles.

Seborrhea: Increased discharge of sebum, the oily secretion of the sebaceous glands of the skin.

Seborrheic dermatitis: Inflammation of the skin sometimes associated with seborrhea.

Shaking palsy: Older, popular term, used in James Parkinson's time, for the specific disorder now called Parkinson's disease or paralysis agitans (see above).

Sleeping sickness: Popular term used during the 1920s and 1930s to refer to encephalitis lethargica (see above). (Another commonly known disease also called sleeping sickness is caused by a parasite transmitted to man and cattle by the bite of the tsetse fly. This disease is limited to Central Africa.)

Solanaceous alkaloids: Bitter-tasting alkaline substances extracted from plants of the family Solanaceae; among them are the botanical drugs atropine, scopolamine, and hyoscyamine.

Stereotactic surgery: Surgical technique for operating deep in the brain without opening the brain and without direct visualization of the site of operation. A long needle-like instrument attached to a frame bolted temporarily to the skull is passed into the brain at angles that are calculated, based on anatomical landmarks, to bring it to a predetermined target. This technique makes it possible to produce very small lesions deep in the brain with considerable precision and minimal injury to the brain.

Striatum: Short for corpus striatum (see above).

Substantia nigra: Anatomical term (from the Latin, meaning black substance) referring to a darkly pigmented area in the upper brainstem that can be seen on visual inspection of specimens of human and primate brains. Substantia nigra cells contain both pigment granules and large amounts of dopamine.

Thalamotomy: Operation, done by stereotactic surgery (see above), in which a small region of the thalamus is destroyed to relieve tremor and rigidity in parkinsonism and other conditions.

Thalamus: Anatomical term designating a mass of gray matter centrally placed deep near the base of the brain. It serves as a major relay station for impulses traveling from the spinal cord and cerebellum to the cerebral cortex.

Tremor: Regular rhythmic to-and-fro involuntary movement affecting a limb, the head, or the entire body.

Tryptophan: One of the nine "essential" amino acids necessary for human nutrition; it is also the metabolic precursor of serotonin, an important chemical messenger in the corpus striatum (see above).

Tyrosine: An amino acid occurring in nature and a normal component of the diet; it is a precursor in the synthesis of dopamine and adrenaline.

Vomiting center: Anatomical and physiological term referring to an area of the medulla oblongata where several clusters of nerve cells initiate and coordinate the act of vomiting.

Von Economo's encephalitis: Another name for encephalitis lethargica (see above). The Viennese neurologist Constantin von Economo is given credit for first recognizing and describing the disorder.

Subject Index